Easy Health Care for Your Horse

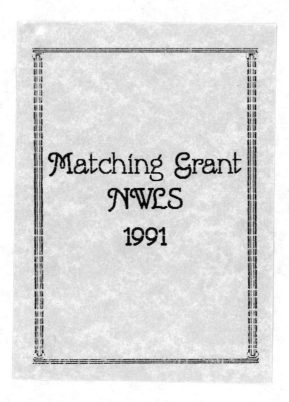

Matching Grant
NWLS
1991

Easy Health Care for Your *Horse*

A Veterinarian's Approach to Prevention Management, and Care

Carin A. Smith, D.V.M.

Illustrations by Heather Lowe
Photographs by Jay Bender

PRENTICE
HALL PRESS
EQUESTRIAN
BOOKS

New York London Toronto Sydney Tokyo Singapore

DISCLAIMER

The author has made every possible effort to ensure that the information contained in this book is accurate. Nonetheless, medicine is a constantly changing field and each case is treated differently depending on individual circumstances. Always consult a veterinarian about your horse's health care and ask for specific instructions about any illness or injury that occurs.

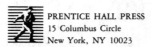 PRENTICE HALL PRESS
15 Columbus Circle
New York, NY 10023

Copyright © 1991 by Dr. Carin A. Smith

PRENTICE HALL PRESS and colophons are registered trademarks
of Simon & Schuster Inc.

Library of Congress Cataloging-in-Publication Data

Smith, Carin A.
    Easy health care for your horse / by Carin A. Smith ;
illustrations by Heather Lowe: photographs by Jay Bender.
        p.   cm.
    ISBN 0-13-223918-3
    1. Horses.   2. Horses—Health.   3. Horses—Diseases.—I. Title.
SF285.3.S65   1991
    636.1'089—dc20   90-24441
                                                                CIP

Designed by Richard Oriolo

Manufactured in the United States of America

10 9 8 7 6 5 4 3 2 1

First Edition 1991

For all horse lovers
and their veterinarians

Contents

Chapter 7. Care of Feet and Hooves 117

Chapter 8. Injuries and Lameness 137

Chapter 9. The Sick Horse 177

Introduction

Easy Health Care for Your Horse is a book for all horse owners, whether new to the world of horses or experienced equestrians. If you're a beginner, you'll love the basic information that is presented in a commonsense manner. Those of you who are more experienced will finally find a nonbiased discussion of alternative methods of therapy, nutritional supplements, new ideas about deworming, and much more.

You'll find the facts you need to know to keep your horse healthy. Starting with a discussion of housing and diet, a complete health program is described, including vaccinations, deworming, and care of teeth and feet. You'll find more up-to-date information here than exists in any other health care book. Does your horse need to be vaccinated against botulism or Potomac horse fever? Should your horse have acupuncture for that chronic sore back problem? After reading this book, you will be able to make intelligent decisions on every aspect of horse health care.

You will spend less money on emergency vet bills when you take the preventive health care approach that is emphasized here. You'll be prepared for unexpected problems, though, with the sections on injuries, lameness, and the sick horse. Read through those chapters before an emergency arises, then use the book as a quick reference when you need help.

This is not a book about how to be your own veterinarian. That kind of expertise takes years of study. Instead, you'll learn how to best utilize your veterinarian, to know when you need help, and to make the most of that assistance.

All horse owners and riders get their fill of advice from people who claim to be experts. While this book does contain suggestions, my goal is to present information so that you can come to your own conclusions about what is best for your horse. It's your obligation to be as informed as possible and to work with your veterinarian to achieve your goals—who knows, next year might bring yet another new vaccine or another new treatment for arthritis. Using this book and the additional sources listed in the appendix will prepare you to evaluate any new ideas in equine health care.

You and your horse have access to the most advanced health care in the world. Take advantage of the knowledge, expertise, and medical care that can help your horse reach his full potential.

Easy Health
Care for Your
Horse

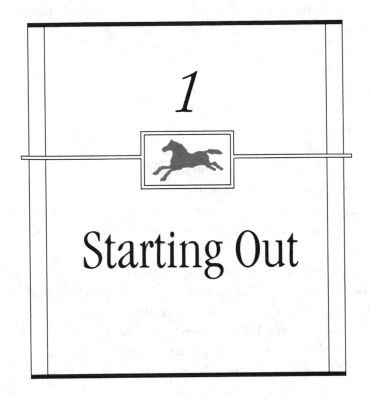

1

Starting Out

Communicate with Your Horse!

Why Do Horses Act the Way They Do?

An unruly horse becomes steady under the control of a twitch. A gentle pony throws its head up as a beginning rider attempts to put on its bridle. Your own horse, who usually trots across the pasture at your call, refuses to come near on the day of the vet's appointment.

What do these horses really perceive in each of these situations, and why do they react the way they do? Behaviors that you might attribute to some sixth sense actually are a horse's reaction to a combination of sights, sounds, smells, and touches. Although the horse has the same five senses that you do, he depends on those senses in different ways.

When your horse seems to behave in mysterious ways, put yourself in his place for a while, and imagine what he may be perceiving. It'll help you get your message across much more effectively.

When you are riding or working closely around your horse, remember that touch and verbal commands are more important than sight to the horse. Touching is used to signal affection, and grooming behavior is common among horses. When your horse nuzzles you, he's not just being friendly; he's identifying you by touch and smell.

Using a twitch to control that unruly horse involves touch in a slightly different way; you can see that twitching actually calms most horses. While some think that the twitch works by distraction, studies have shown that the use of the twitch causes release of endorphins, the body's natural painkiller.

Your body language says something to your horse, and his body language tells you something, too. Changes in the position of your horse's body, head, ears, and tail send off clear signals of what he's feeling. His ears may point forward indicating interest, or lie back in a show of aggression. Ears laid flat with the head lowered just indicates a relaxed state of mind. Your horse raises his tail when he's confident or excited, tucks it in to show fear or submission. Soft nickers are signs of familiarity and affection between mares and foals, pasture buddies, or from a horse to its human owner. Snorting or blowing signals alarm or playfulness.

That gentle pony resisted being bridled because the rider raised his hand directly in front of the pony's face. The pony threw its head up simply to try to see what was happening.

What Is In the Eye

The clear cornea covers the front of the eye. Behind the cornea lies the aqueous humor, the fluid that helps hold the eyeball's shape and lubricates the inside of the eye and iris.

The iris is a muscular structure that constricts and expands to change the size of the pupil, an opening that allows more or less light into the back of the eye. The horse's iris comes in a variety of colors, from brown to blue to white. Blue eyes, common in Welsh ponies, have been called "wall eyes" or "china eyes." The white iris is called a "glass eye." Horses with a white iris may have problems in bright light. Some light-colored or spotted horses have spots or patches of a different color in their iris; this is normal.

Have you ever noticed the lump on the upper edge of your horse's iris? The corpora nigra, a projection of the iris, works like a shade to keep out excess light on bright days. Albino horses may have a hypoplastic

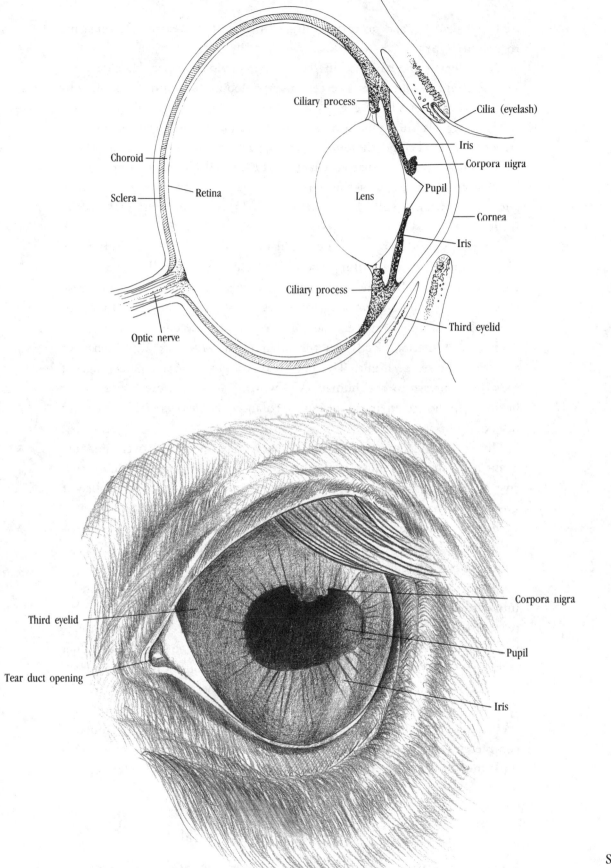

Ciliary process

Cilia (eyelash)

Iris

Corpora nigra

Choroid

Sclera

Retina

Lens

Pupil

Cornea

Iris

Ciliary process

Third eyelid

Optic nerve

Corpora nigra

Third eyelid

Pupil

Tear duct opening

Iris

3

Starting Out

(reduced-size) iris and no corpora nigra, making them extremely sensitive to bright light.

The sclera is the white of the eye that is obvious in people. You can't see the sclera in most horses, except in Appaloosas, which have an obvious rim of white around the eye.

Light travels through the pupil and is refracted by the lens, an oval structure lying behind the pupil opening. The shape of the lens is altered by the ciliary muscles that attach it to the eyeball. Most mammals focus by changing the shape of the lens. The horse's ciliary muscles are weak and the lens fairly stiff. Horses' ability to focus at different distances is limited.

After passing through the lens, light passes through a liquid called the vitreous humor before striking the retina. This layer of cells lying on the back of the eyeball gathers information and sends it through the optic nerve to the brain. There are two types of photoreceptor cell found in the retina, the rods and the cones. The cones provide daytime vision and color discrimination. Rods, on the other hand, are more light sensitive and work better at night. The horse eye contains a high percentage of rods, in contrast to the human eye, which contains more cones. Your horse's superiority in night vision is balanced by a decreased ability to discern color.

Horses, and many other mammals, have one advantage over humans. Their night vision is much better because of the tapetum, a highly reflective area in the back of the eye. The tapetum is what causes the bright green glow you see when shining a light into an animal's eyes at night.

Horses with colored coats but light colored eyes may have slightly less effective night vision because of a smaller tapetum. Cream colored horses (white coat with blue eyes) may not have a tapetum at all.

Horses don't cry, but produce tears continuously in small amounts to lubricate and cleanse the cornea. Irritation of the eye or nose causes more tear production and the overflow runs down the face. The tear duct, which drains tears from the eye into the nose, opens on the inside corner of the eyelid. The duct traverses the nose to open just inside the horse's nostril. If you look carefully, you can see this opening.

Horses have eyelashes on the upper eyelid only. The upper and lower eyelids are lined on the inside with the pink conjunctiva. The conjunctiva completely surrounds the "third eyelid," or nictating membrane. This pink membrane can be seen on the inner, lower corner of each eye.

Equine Eyesight:
How Your Horse Sees the World

While riding along a mountain trail one lazy afternoon, your horse unexpectedly leaps sideways, interrupting your daydreaming. Only after a look around do you notice the dog behind you. Your horse has seen dogs before, so what was the problem?

Easy Health Care
For Your Horse

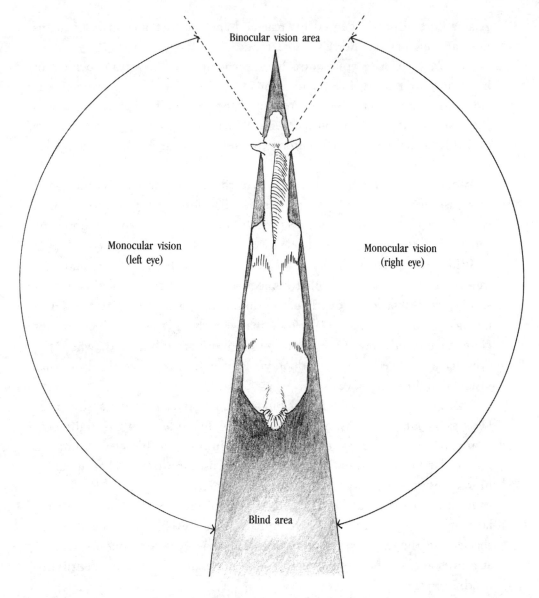

Binocular vision area

Monocular vision
(left eye)

Monocular vision
(right eye)

Blind area

Horses appear to have good eyesight at times, yet spook at what appear to you to be ordinary objects. That's because the horse's eyes function far differently from yours.

Horse eyes developed over time to help this grazing animal to survive. The horse's priority was not clarity of vision, but rather an ability to scan over large areas of the horizon for warning signs from predators. The eyes' placement on the sides of the head provided a large field of view while the horse grazed. The horizontal shape of the pupil helped in seeing a broad lateral view.

While you're riding, your horse can see things that you can't. If a dog sneaks up behind the side of your horse as you ride, your horse may see him while you're obliviously looking ahead. Any unfamiliar moving object appearing in the horse's lateral vision may be cause for nervousness or spooking.

In spite of a broad range of vision, the horse does have some blind spots. Keep these in mind while riding and working around your horse.

5

Starting Out

A small area directly behind his rear end and another just in front of his nose are out of your horse's visual range.

You may surprise your horse by approaching directly from behind or by lifting your hand directly in front of his face. Be sure to stand to the side and let your horse see where your hands are going before you touch those spots outside of his visual field. When you groom your horse's face or apply a twitch, reach up from the side so your horse can see your hand.

While you're riding, remember that the horse cannot see the small area just in front of and under his nose. The jumper sets up for a jump way ahead of time, since at the time he takes off from the ground, the jump itself is out of his field of vision.

While the horse is looking to either side, each eye moves and sees independently in what is called monocular vision. Because of this way of seeing, horses have no depth perception. The horse has to judge depth by the size of an object and by how that size changes as the object moves closer or farther away. Only when he's looking straight ahead, where the eyes have an overlapping field of view, can he see with the binocular vision that humans have.

Changing from monocular to binocular vision can have its surprises. Let's say your horse has spotted a bush by his side with his right eye. You turn him to the right, and the bush "jumps," in his view, from the monocular field of vision to a binocular, focused position. That apparent movement may be enough to make him spook.

Another disadvantage of that broad field of view is the horse's relative lack of focusing ability. Most mammals focus by changing the shape of the lens in the eye. Experts believe that equine eyes have one focus level at all distances. The horse uses the sense of smell as an aid in identifying nearby objects.

Color vision in the horse is the subject of controversy. Does the horse see color, or only differentiate between shades of gray? We'll probably never know for sure, but it is certain that the horse's ability to differentiate color is far inferior to yours. Probably the horse sees shades and brightness more than the actual colors that you can see.

Inside the Ear

The ear consists of inner, middle, and outer parts. The horse's external ear has a large funnel shape, which collects sounds from the outside world. The thin tympanic membrane separating the external and middle ears vibrates in response to sound, sending it through the middle ear. The three auditory ossicles (bones) lying within the tympanic cavity of the middle ear help to amplify sound. Sound vibrates through the middle ear into the inner ear. Within the inner ear lies the osseous labyrinth, a

Easy Health Care
For Your Horse

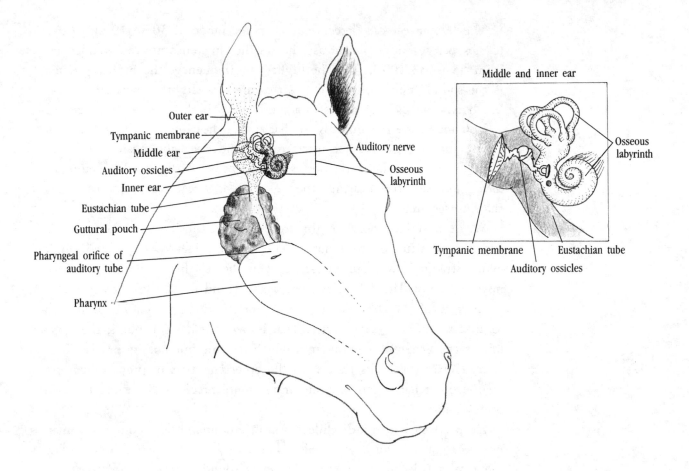

Middle and inner ear

Outer ear

Tympanic membrane

Middle ear

Auditory ossicles

Inner ear

Eustachian tube

Guttural pouch

Pharyngeal orifice of
auditory tube

Pharynx

Auditory nerve

Osseous
labyrinth

Osseous
labyrinth

Tympanic membrane

Auditory ossicles

Eustachian tube

curlicue of delicate bones that are the receivers of sound. The auditory nerve, lying within this structure, sends information to the brain where it is interpreted as sound.

The tympanic cavity of the middle ear connects to the pharynx (back of the throat) by the eustachian or auditory tube. This tube has a slitlike opening at the back of the pharynx that helps equalize pressure between the tympanic cavity and the outside world.

In the horse, the auditory tubes have unusual extensions, the guttural pouches. With no known function, these pouches go relatively unnoticed unless they become infected. They connect the auditory tube to the back of the pharynx.

How Horses Hear

Your horse grazes quietly out in the pasture and seems oblivious to your presence near the barn. But when you scoop a can full of grain out of the barrel, his head pops up, instantly alert to the prospect of breakfast.

Horses have an extremely good sense of hearing. Studies of many different animals' hearing has shown that the horse's hearing has more similarities to yours than it has differences.

The human ear can detect sounds in the range of 30 to 19,000 hertz (cycles per second); in contrast, horses' hearing encompasses frequencies from 55 to 33,500 hertz. The higher the frequency, the higher pitched is the sound. You can hear sounds that are of a slightly lower frequency, but horses can pick up noises in a considerably higher frequency range.

You may have the impression that horses' hearing is more acute than yours. Just because a horse reacts to a sound does not mean that it has heard more than you have; horses startle easily. Although other animals have more sensitive hearing, they're much less reactive to those sounds than horses are.

While a sudden noise might arouse your curiosity, it could mean a threatening situation to a horse. You might prefer to study and think about strange new occurrences, but your horse's first reaction is to flee now and think later. That is the reason behind his "spook" reaction.

In spite of the attentive appearance of the horse's ears, his ability to localize sound isn't very precise. That is, when it hears a sound, the horse knows the general direction from which it came but not its precise location. Horses share this trait with the other creatures of prey. Predators, on the other hand, can pinpoint much more precisely the exact location of a sound.

Keep all this in mind while working around horses. Your horse may not hear you talking if your voice is at a very low frequency (low pitch). He may spook due to a high frequency sound that you can't hear, or simply due to a sound that he perceives as threatening.

The tone of voice you use around your horse tells him a great deal. An uncertain tone invites him to ignore you or disobey. A definite and steady voice tells him that you really mean what you say.

Most horses respond to particular sounds in specific ways. The soothing tones of Mozart played in the barn may help to quiet a nervous horse, while loud rock and roll might get the whole barn stirred up. Some horses prefer particular types of music. Try playing different tunes in your barn, and see if there are any changes in your horse's attitude.

Noise Phobias

Many noises are particularly irritating or frightening to horses. Such noises may interfere with their ability to function in a given situation. The show horse that rears at the sound of clippers or the racehorse that becomes unmanageable around a large noisy crowd both suffer from noise phobias, or unreasonable fears.

You can reduce your horse's noise phobia by gradually conditioning the horse to the sound. One study showed that clipper fear was significantly reduced by having a running set of clippers placed outside horses' stalls each time they were fed.

The horse that spooks at the sounds of a large crowd of people may be helped by playing a tape of those sounds at low volume in the barn while he's relaxed and quiet. Gradually increase the volume as he becomes accustomed to the noise.

Pay close attention when your horse spooks "unnecessarily" at a particular sound. With a little thought, you may be able to prevent the reaction next time.

Your Horse's Good Taste

From watermelons to beer to peppermint candies, every horse has his favorite treat. Some love apples but shun carrots, while others will eat almost anything you offer. Have you ever wondered just what horses can taste, and whether they experience taste the same way that you do?

Can horses pick out the most nutritious feeds by their sense of taste? Is cribbing a sign of a lack of some particular mineral in your horse's diet? There are many unanswered questions in the area of equine taste. There are also many known facts that will help you to keep your horse healthy and happy.

Since your horse can't tell you about his likes and dislikes, the only way to discern his tastes is by observing his actions. But the reasons behind your horse's eating behavior may be far different from what you'd like to believe.

There is no question that horses can experience taste. Salty, sweet, and bitter are all differentiated. Your horse licks his salt block, eagerly munches an apple, or shuns the scrumptious-looking pile of grain with medicine sneakily mixed in. The sense of smell is closely tied in with taste, and the horse may shun that medicated sweet feed even before he tastes it.

Horses cannot pick out the more nutritious feed when offered a choice. They do not prefer higher-calorie hay over a lower-calorie batch if both are clean and of good quality. The same goes for hay that is higher in needed vitamins or minerals. Your horse may shun moldy hay or pick through carefully for clean wisps. Still, don't count on your horse's taste to tell you whether his feed is adequate or to protect him from eating feeds that might endanger his health.

Horses occasionally sense what's bad for them, as seen in the pastured horse's tendency to separate his grazing area from his manure pile. Only when conditions are crowded or the grazing area sparse will he nibble around his own waste.

Similarly, your horse may shun poisonous plants due to their unpleasant taste or because of his preference for tastier pasture grasses. Yet dangerous plants don't all taste bad, and a horse can't associate sickness with what he ate hours before. If the pasture is grazed down, the horse will eat whatever is available.

Your horse might prefer certain grains over others. Most horses prefer oats over corn or barley. The horse's love of grain can lead to trouble if you accidentally leave the grain bin open. Too much of a good thing can be very dangerous, and the horse doesn't know when to stop.

Many show horses are particular about the taste of their water, which can become a problem for the traveling competitor. You can fool your horse by lightly flavoring the water at home with vinegar, sweetened Kool-aid, sugar, or mint. Then use the same flavor in the "new" water.

Horses cannot adjust their eating behavior to compensate for vitamin deficiencies. For example, a deficiency in calcium does not lead to a hunger for that mineral. There is no inborn sense of vitamin and mineral balance, and no way for the horse to determine the vitamin or mineral content of his feed. One exception is the horse's natural hunger for salt. When deprived of salt and then offered a salt block, the horse will have an increased appetite for the mineral.

What, then, is the explanation for odd eating and chewing behaviors, such as wood chewing? It's an extremely rare case that truly has a nutritional deficiency. Most often, boredom or a lack of roughage is the problem. Horses are natural grazers, and if not provided with enough hay to satisfy their chewing needs, they will chew on whatever is available. Meals offered twice or three times a day might provide adequate nutrition, but the horse's natural tendency to chew on something all day long is still there. Horses fed a pellet ration are particularly susceptible to wood chewing. Plenty of activity and a large turnout area might help to prevent problems from occurring.

Another odd taste habit sometimes seen is an addiction to salt. Horses with this problem literally consume their salt block in a matter of days. In these cases, loose salt must be given in daily measured amounts to supply the horse's needs.

You can use your horse's sweet tooth to fool him into taking otherwise shunned medicine. First you may have to do some experimenting to discover which flavor he prefers and which flavor masks the taste of the drug; try using molasses, applesauce, or peanut butter.

You can use bad-tasting substances to advantage. Have you ever had a horse that just wouldn't leave a wrap alone? You can use homemade concoctions or commercial products to frighten away your horse's taste buds. Tabasco sauce is a classic, but an occasional horse ignores that fiery warning, spurring its owner on to further inventions. Be careful not to use anything that may harm the horse or burn its lips. Put the product on the wrap only, not on the horse's skin or hair.

Use your horse's good and bad taste preferences to your advantage. Learning more about what he likes will make life easier for you both.

Easy Health Care
For Your Horse

Choose a Veterinarian
You Can Trust

Your first decision about horse care will be that of choosing a veterinarian. How will you decide on a veterinarian for your horse? The choosing of a veterinarian can't be done with just a perusal of the Yellow Pages. Perhaps you've just begun to look for a veterinarian, or maybe you're thinking of switching doctors. Take your time and be sure that you're comfortable with your decision. With some helpful guidelines, you and your veterinarian can begin a close relationship of understanding and trust.

Where and How to Look

Ask your neighbors and fellow riders whom they use, and why they may dislike one veterinarian or prefer another. Your friend with the brood mare farm is thrilled with her vet, a reproductive expert, but that doctor won't be much help to your hunter-jumper gelding.

Your local horse clubs, stables, and breeders are other good sources of information. You'll find that every veterinarian will be both liked and disliked by a certain number of people. What you're looking for are the names that come up most often.

You can use the phone directory to get a list of hospitals and veterinarians in your area, but don't stop there. Many of the best hospitals have only a one-line ad, while other less respectable operations may buy a full page. Make a list from the phone directory, and use that as a base from which to start your search.

Before you actually begin looking, you'll need to answer some important questions. What aspects of veterinary care are the most important to you? Availability and location? Getting the same doctor each time? Cost? Expertise in a particular area of medicine or surgery? Hospital facilities? Horsemanship? Personality?

You might choose a general practitioner or a specialist. General practitioners in rural areas will work on all types of animals. In other areas, you'll have the choice of mobile equine veterinarians and veterinary specialists ranging from surgeons to ophthalmologists.

Some veterinarians will cater to particular types of horse owners. The show horse, race horse, and endurance horse have unique problems, and a veterinarian who's aware of them can help you in countless ways. If your vet participates in the same sport that you do, that's even better.

A larger or specialized hospital might be appropriate for larger farms or for riders involved in competition at the higher levels. The expertise and care provided by Dr. Impressive are optimal, with several specialists on staff. However, a multiple-doctor practice often means you'll be dealing with a different veterinarian each time. Yet choosing the least expensive vet for routine health care might leave you stranded when your horse has a complicated colic in the middle of the night.

Imagine the scenario: "Yes, I usually use Doctor Cheapest, but he doesn't answer the phone at night. Can you come look at my horse right now?" Dr. Good, who hasn't the slightest idea who you are and figures you probably can't pay the bill anyhow, tells you it'll probably wait until morning.

Evaluating Potential Veterinarians

Once you've got a few names, visit the veterinary hospitals and meet the doctors and their staff. If your choice is a mobile vet, call or stop by the office.

Find out how the veterinary service is run. Are appointments required? How far ahead must they be scheduled? If there is more than one veterinarian, find out whether one will be assigned to you. Be sure you're comfortable with them all, though. One doctor can't be on call all the time, and you may get any of them for an out-of-hours emergency.

Watch the interactions among receptionists, technicians, doctors, and clients. Is everyone friendly, working together as a team? Are the staff comfortable around horses? Are clients treated courteously and with respect? Are procedures explained to the clients in words they can understand?

Are the hospital and the veterinary trucks clean and neat? Are the stalls picked out, and water buckets full? Is an isolation stall available for infectious cases?

Does the hospital have written handouts explaining their policies, their recommended health program, and other common procedures? Does the veterinarian set up a yearly health program for each horse? Is a regular newsletter sent to clients? Do the doctors conduct seminars for their clients, or hold classes through the local colleges?

While everyone wants to save money, save the question of cost until you've narrowed your choices to a few good veterinarians. Most veterinarians fall in between the two extremes of Dr. Cheapest and Dr. Impressive. Once you've chosen someone you like, you can discuss your personal financial situation and ways to economize without harming your horse's health.

The Horse Owner on a Budget

There are many ways you can economize and still receive the best possible care for your horse. Discuss your financial situation with your veterinarian. Being on a budget shouldn't mean sacrificing your horse's health.

If your vet works out of a clinic or hospital, you can bring your horse there rather than pay a trip fee. If you don't have a trailer, perhaps a friend will lend you one, or even load your horse with hers for the annual deworming and other regular visits.

Many veterinarians will give a discounted trip fee if you organize your neighbors and schedule all routine work for one day of the week. Ask your vet about vaccination or deworming "clinics." These are held at one particular stable or in a small town that doesn't have a full time veterinarian.

No veterinarian will make a diagnosis or prescribe treatments over the phone. We're required *by law* to have an "established patient–doctor relationship." That relationship doesn't mean, for example, that we dispensed bute to you for a similar problem last year; it means we see you and your horse regularly.

Tell your veterinarian if you are able and willing to give injections or do treatments yourself. Be sure that you practice any new techniques while the veterinarian is there for help and advice. Carefully follow the vet's instructions and advice on how to proceed. Trying to save money by adopting the "wait-and-see" approach to problems won't save you money in the end. Get that cut looked at while it's fresh, and it'll cost a lost less to treat than an old, infected wound.

If you plan to do your own vaccinations and paste dewormings, you should still discuss a health program with your vet. Vaccination and deworming recommendations are changing every day. Find out what's optimal for your horse, rather than taking a guess.

You will save money by thinking ahead about a health plan for your horse. Your horse's health program is a yearly schedule of dewormings, vaccinations, dental care, trimming, and shoeing. It is a plan of your horse's feeding, feed supplements, exercise schedule, and shelter. Your goal is to reduce the costs of treating problems by preventing them in the first place. You'll be able to anticipate costs rather than guess at emergency bills. The result is a healthy horse and a happy owner.

When Should You Switch Veterinarians?

Have you ever felt doubts about your veterinarian? If you have, you're not alone. Personality conflicts, overwork and exhaustion, and simple mistakes do occur. When is one more mistake too many? When do you decide that, no matter how hard you try, you just can't see eye to eye with your veterinarian?

First, try to narrow down the problem. Is it the way a particular case was handled, or is it a personality conflict? Are you uncomfortable with the way your vet handles your horse? Is the vet always late? Be sure that the lines of communication are open. Have you discussed the problem? Talking it out may not be easy, but is often the best solution in the long run. Once you have cleared the air you can get on to a fresh start. Maybe all you need is a second opinion on a case. If so, discuss the situation rather than simply taking your horse to another vet.

"Dr. Good, I'm really concerned that old Joe isn't recuperating as fast as I'd expected. Can we have Dr. Specialist look at him?" Dr. Good replies, "Sure. I'll mail the X rays over and give her a call to explain what we've done so far."

By having your doctor work *with* another, your horse comes out the winner, and you don't have to pay to have tests repeated unnecessarily. No good veterinarian takes offense about a request for a second opinion; it's part of our work atmosphere.

If you've talked out the problem and nothing has changed, then maybe it's time to switch. Once you've decided, stick with your new choice. Switching around from vet to vet doesn't help your horse, and it may convince other doctors in the area not to take you on as a client. Be sure to have copies of your records sent to your new veterinarian so your horse's health care will continue uninterrupted.

The Veterinary
Prepurchase Examination

What It Is, and Why You Need It

The day you brought your new horse home was one of the happiest days of spring. Turned out in his new pasture, the bay gelding romped about as if he'd always been there. For the first few weeks of riding, everything went smoothly, as you two got to know each other. But after a month of intense training, the gelding became mildly yet persistently lame. Who's responsible for the vet bills?

Your new yearling filly has impeccable bloodlines. Her former owner assured you that she had a history of consistently winning halter ribbons. Now that you've brought her home, though, you find that the quiet filly you bought has changed dramatically; she's absolutely unmanageable. Can you get your money back?

These situations could easily be avoided. Isn't it better to discover a horse's faults *before* you own it, rather than afterward?

While you're looking for that dream horse, you'll need someone to help you to be sure you're making the right choice. Once you take your horse home, you can concentrate on having fun.

14

Easy Health Care
For Your Horse

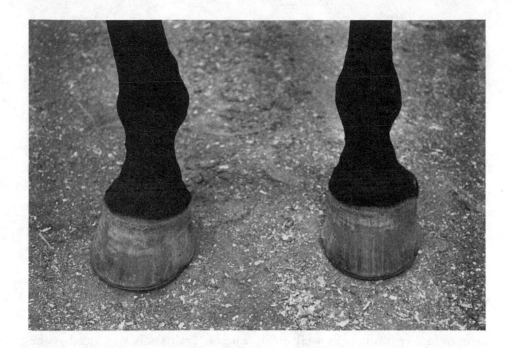

The "prepurchase exam" is done on any horse you're considering buying, to evaluate both the horse's health and its suitability for the work you intend. It is not a pass/fail exam, but an evaluation of the horse's strengths and weaknesses. With this knowledge, you can make an informed decision on whether or not the horse is the one you want.

"But," you say, "this horse is going for a bargain price and my trainer assures me that he's just what I'm looking for!"
Will your trainer pay the veterinary bills and cost of upkeep? A horse that's unsuitable for your use will cost as much to feed and house as one that's just right—so think of this exam as an investment.

Your veterinarian can work within your budget, knowing your priorities, to give you a helpful evaluation of your prospect. When a more detailed examination or further tests are indicated, you can decide whether you want to continue with the exam or try for a different horse.

Before the Vet's Exam

The veterinary exam should be done after you've done a little work yourself. The veterinarian will not answer specific questions on a horse's ability to jump five-foot fences, or a pony's suitability for your seven-year old child.

The person who will be riding the horse should take him out to be sure he's able to do the work intended. Get a trainer's help if you aren't sure; a trainer or other knowledgeable horse person will also help you decide whether the animal is worth the purchase price. The veterinarian's role is only to evaluate the horse's health and physical condition as they relate to its intended use.

Once you've picked out a horse you really like, call your veterinarian for an appointment. As the buyer, you are the one who must request and pay for the exam. It is a legal conflict of interest for the seller's vet to do this exam. (An exception might be made if the seller agrees to make the entire medical record available to the buyer. This could work for or against the buyer, depending on the circumstances).

Set aside a few hours for the exam. Spend some time explaining to your vet just what you're looking for in a horse. A child's pony can get by with a minor arthritis problem, but an eventing prospect must be sound enough to take an intensive training program. Also, be sure to tell the doctor about all the possible uses you envision for this horse. If you're looking at an eventing mare but are also considering breeding her, a reproductive workup as well as an athletic evaluation will need to be performed.

How the Exam is Done

Each doctor will conduct the prepurchase exam in a different way, but they all will perform a methodical and thorough examination. Keep in mind that this procedure varies among veterinarians and among any one vet's clients. For illustrative purposes, we'll follow one veterinarian through a typical prepurchase exam.

The examination starts on the horse at rest. First, the veterinarian stands back, getting an overall impression of how the horse looks, noting any obvious problems. Then a closer, head-to-toe inspection is done.

Is the animal over- or underweight? Does he look alert and healthy? Is his overall conformation acceptable? Areas of questionable appearance are noted for further evaluation.

The horse's conformation can have a direct effect on his ability to perform certain functions; some faults may be immediately disqualifying, but most simply predispose the horse to particular problems.

Certain uses also predispose the horse to particular types of problems. For example, a horse that is back at the knee might be predisposed to chip fractures. Cow hocks (turned in as viewed from behind) predispose the horse to bone spavin. Straight pasterns cause increased concussion of the lower leg and foot, predisposing the animal to navicular disease or ankle problems.

Combining these conformation faults with an activity that puts extra stress on those areas will increase the likelihood of a problem sometime down the road. Once you are aware of these predispositions, you can take steps to prevent problems in the future, or you can decide that it's not

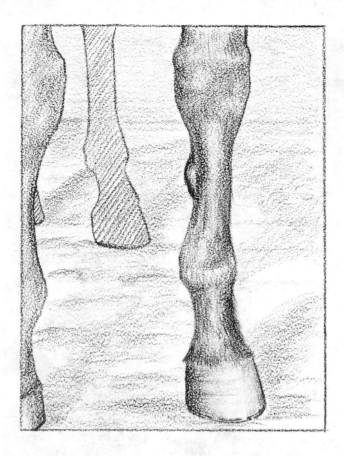

worth the effort. Remember that perfectly conformed horses are rarities, and a conformation fault in itself may not remove a horse from consideration.

Blemishes must be differentiated from real problems. A blemish is a defect that does not affect the intended use. For example, an old splint could be a blemish, while a new, sore splint might be an unsoundness.

The horse's eyes are viewed with an ophthalmoscope. Previous bouts with "moon blindness," an inflammatory condition of the eye, may leave telltale signs.

The horse's approximate age is determined by the appearance of the teeth. Cribbers, or horses that chew and suck on wood, will be readily apparent from the excessive wear on the incisors. (Although it is not the veterinarian's responsibility to discover all the horse's vices, you will be told if there are physical signs of them).

The veterinarian will note the presence of any malocclusions of the teeth. These include "parrot mouth" (overhanging upper jaw), "sow mouth" (protruding lower jaw), and "wave mouth" (uneven wear of the molars). These are problems that will require continual care. Consider the hereditary aspect of these conditions in breeding animals.

Abnormalities of the skin are also noted. Tumors such as melanoma, sometimes found in gray horses, might be spotted.

Your veterinarian will carefully palpate the horse's back and all four

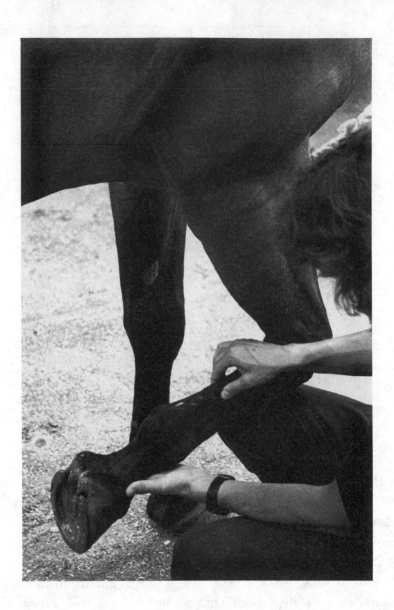

legs. Deep pressure along the spine will reveal a sore back. Swellings in the soft tissues of the legs will be readily apparent. All joints are manipulated to check for normal, full range of motion.

The feet are picked out and the hoof wall, sole, and frog are checked for normal growth and symmetry. Signs of founder may include a widened white line on the bottom of the foot. A dubbed (excessively worn) toe might indicate dragging of the foot or pain in the heel area because the horse tries to land toe first with every stride. Hoof testers are applied to detect soreness.

The cardiovascular system is examined at rest, and again after exercise. A horse's fitness can be gauged by the time it takes for the pulse to drop after exercise.

The heart and lungs are auscultated with a stethoscope to pick up any abnormal sounds. Heart murmurs are not uncommon in horses, and if present are evaluated for significance. Many benign (insignificant) murmurs disappear with exercise.

Easy Health Care
For Your Horse

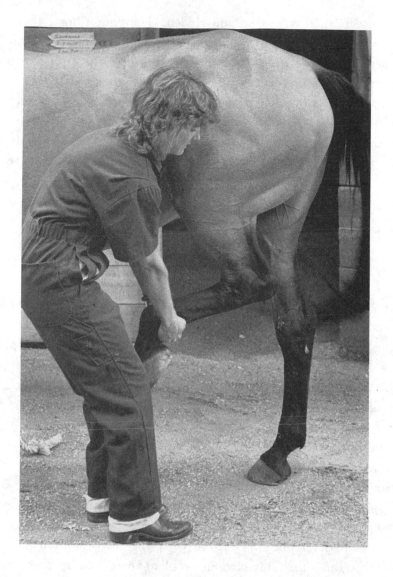

If there is any question of a problem, special tests such as an electrocardiogram (ECG) or echocardiography (ultrasonic evaluation of the heart) are run. Some insurance companies now require an ECG on all horses insured over a certain value.

The lungs are evaluated for any abnormal sounds, such as those suggestive of allergic problems. A bag placed over the horse's nose will force deeper breathing and help to accentuate any abnormal sounds.

The horse is evaluated moving at the walk and trot, in a line, in circles, on hard and soft ground, and sometimes on hills. Lameness, interference, or unusual ways of going can be seen. Several aspects of the horse's movement are considered, including stride length, symmetry, the arc of the foot as it passes through the stride, and how the foot lands. Any abnormality will tip off the veterinarian to areas of soreness.

Flexion tests are performed to accentuate any soreness that may be present. The leg is picked up while one or more joints are held in flexion for a minute before the horse is trotted off.

The horse is then tacked up and ridden. The young horse that is not yet being ridden is turned out into a large exercise area or round pen. Keeping the findings of the physical exam in mind, the veterinarian pays special attention to problems that might cause lameness.

Next, further testing may be discussed and undertaken. Your veterinarian could recommend several different procedures after the basic physical exam is done. Whether or not you decide to have these performed depends on your priorities, budget, expectations for the future of your horse, and the findings of the exam up to this point.

Special Procedures:
Requirement or Rip-off?

Your veterinarian may recommend laboratory tests as part of the workup. These include a complete blood count, fecal exam for parasites, drug screening, and serum chemistries. (See "Laboratory Tests" in chapter 9, *The Sick Horse.*)

Racehorses may receive an endoscopic exam. A flexible fiberoptic tube is inserted into the nose to view the throat area. The veterinarian looks for abnormalities in the larynx and trachea.

A mare being purchased as a breeding prospect requires special evaluation of her reproductive tract. The breeding stallion will also need a complete fertility exam.

Radiographs (X rays) are commonly taken during prepurchase exams. What areas need to be radiographed? One opinion is that certain areas ought to be radiographed no matter what the physical exam suggests. Another thought is that only obvious problem areas need be radiographed.

Many radiographic findings are ambiguous. Radiographic findings such as bone changes on an X ray must be correlated with the physical exam to determine their significance. For example, veterinarians frequently hear a request for radiographic evaluation of the navicular bones. There are a certain number of horses that have "abnormal" radiographs of their navicular bones but are not lame. Conversely, many horses with clinical signs of navicular disease have very little in the way of radiographic changes.

You might consider an ultrasonic examination of the horse's tendons. Ultrasound will help the veterinarian evaluate questionable areas of the tendons or ligaments in the lower leg.

Common sense should dictate just how far to go with special procedures. Lack of any testing at all could leave several questions unanswered, but doing every possible test available is cost restrictive and carries some risk. The cost and risk must be weighed against the the benefit of doing the test and the probability that the procedure will yield useful information.

Decision Time

After the workup is complete, you'll sit down with your veterinarian to summarize what you've discovered. The prepurchase exam done by your veterinarian might be similar to the one described here, or it may differ in many ways. In any case, the important point is that the horse must be examined thoroughly and to your satisfaction.

The veterinarian only verifies the horse's condition at the time of the exam. There are no guarantees for the future. However, after all this you'll be thoroughly acquainted with your new companion and will be better prepared for whatever the future may bring.

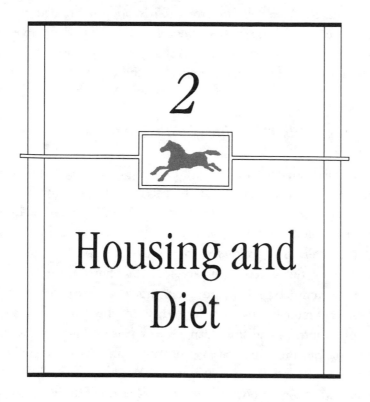

2

Housing and Diet

Horse Housing

Where Will Your Horse Live?

Housing for horses is as varied as the people who own them. Whether you've kept your horse in the same place for years, or are looking for a new pasture or stable, some important considerations must be kept in mind.

Safety is your first concern when making any decision about your horse's housing. Whether you use a barn or pasture, all structures from fence posts and gates to doors and walls must be set firmly in place. Temporary repairs of broken parts with a strand of baling wire won't hold up against a frightened horse, and you'll have a wreck on your hands.

Fencing may be made of wood, wire, pipe, concrete, plastic, or rubber. Any fence material can be dangerous if it's not maintained properly. If you must have a wire fence, choose smooth wire over barbed. Even smooth wire can cut your horse, though, so tie bright orange ribbons at intervals along the fence, or use electric fencing on the top wire.

Barns, Stalls, and Paddocks

A stall or small paddock has the advantage of keeping your horse close at hand; there's no chasing around the pasture after an unwilling mount. Daily cleaning is essential, and your horse will need regular feeding times. An hour or more of daily exercise, either by turnout or riding, is a must.

Barns can offer what appears to be comfortable protection against the weather. During the winter, you can close your horse tight inside. Without adequate ventilation, though, your horse is better off out in that storm. As the temperature and humidity in the barn rise, so do the numbers of airborne organisms. Dangerous levels of dust, molds, bacteria, and ammonia can build up. Even a healthy horse will become sick, and allergic horses are absolutely miserable.

Provide ventilation by opening windows that don't allow a direct breeze on the horse. During bad weather when these are closed, ventilation is still necessary. The barn should have openings both at ground level and near the top for good air flow. No drafts should blow on the horses, though.

When there's a choice, pick sliding stall doors over ones that swing out. Latches should have smooth edges with safety catches to prevent your horse from accidentally turning himself loose. Feed and water containers should be smooth and securely fastened. Check for loose or protruding nails and boards.

Boarding stables are the best choice for many people. You can choose one where you don't have any work except to come out and ride your horse, or economize by doing some of the feeding or cleaning yourself. Quality of care can vary widely, so be sure to investigate thoroughly. After you get several recommendations, visit the barns, have a look around, and talk to the people who board their horses there.

Look for clean stalls, a lack of safety hazards, and good quality feed. Choose a stable that offers a turnout service for your horse on days when you don't ride. No horse should be left in a stall all day.

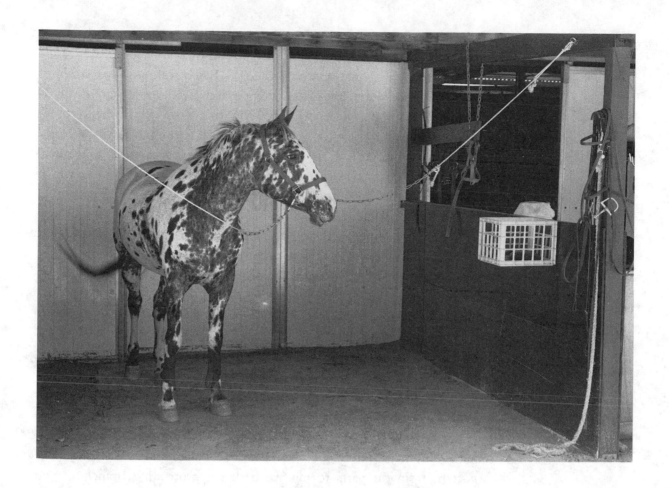

Stall Bedding

Your choices of stall bedding range from peanut hulls to straw. Availability and cost have the greatest effect on your decision, but there are health considerations as well.

Why use bedding at all? Floors in a barn may be dirt, sand, concrete, or rubber mats. All of these can be very abrasive to the horse's legs when he lies down. Some become slippery and dangerous when wet. In addition to providing a cushion, bedding absorbs urine, so that it can be removed regularly.

Remove all soiled bedding each day. Every week or two, take out all the bedding and thoroughly clean the floor beneath. This deep cleaning helps prevent a dangerous buildup of ammonia in the air.

Straw is a good bedding material. Good quality straw creates very little dust, provides good cushioning, and is easy to clean. However, straw isn't as absorbent as some other materials, and it can become moldy and dusty.

Wood shavings or sawdust can work well, too. Their absorbency is quite good, but they tend to be dusty. Good-quality wood shavings are less dusty than poor-quality straw, though. Black walnut wood shavings are poisonous to horses. Be sure that your supplier knows that the shavings will be used for horse bedding, and that you know what type of wood is contained in them.

Shredded newspaper can be obtained cheaply in some areas. It's absorbent and soft, but can become very messy. Avoid using newspaper if your horse eats his bedding.

You can use peanut hulls, corn husks, or rice hulls for bedding. They don't absorb moisture well, and are a potential hazard if the horse eats them. Rice hulls are light, dusty, and easily inhaled. Don't use them for young horses, those with respiratory problems, or horses that lie down a lot.

Keeping Your Horse on Pasture

Pasture might be the best place for your horse if you want a minimal workload. With good pasture, you won't have to feed every day, and your horse is always turned out for exercise. You still have a little work, though. Check for poisonous plants, hidden holes, and items long since forgotten, from car parts to logs with sharp, protruding branches. You must provide daily fresh water all year round. Your horse cannot get enough water from eating snow in the winter.

Consult your county extension agent for advice on seeding, fertilization, weed control, and insect problems. (Look in the phone book under county government, department of agriculture, or agriculture agent.) Keep weeds down to an acceptable level with good fertilization and grazing management. Clipping in the spring, before seeds form, reduces the spread of weeds. If you use herbicides or insecticides, be sure to use a product that's labeled safe for pastures.

Horses kept at pasture will need shelter from the weather. This shelter needn't be fancy, but it must offer protection from sun, wind, rain, and snow. A group of trees does the job in areas with mild winters. In other places, a three-sided shed facing away from the wind is adequate.

Horses kept outdoors year-round will develop a thick protective coat that keeps them comfortable through snowy winters. Blankets are not necessary for horses that live outside all the time. However, if you want to keep a show coat on your horse, then you must provide a barn or stall shelter, and keep the horse blanketed to protect him from the cold.

Manure pickup is as important on pasture as in a stall or paddock. If you leave manure where it lies, you run the risk of a gradual, dangerous buildup of parasite eggs in the pasture. Also, since horses will avoid grazing around "roughs," or areas of manure piles, much of the pasture

Easy Health Care
For Your Horse

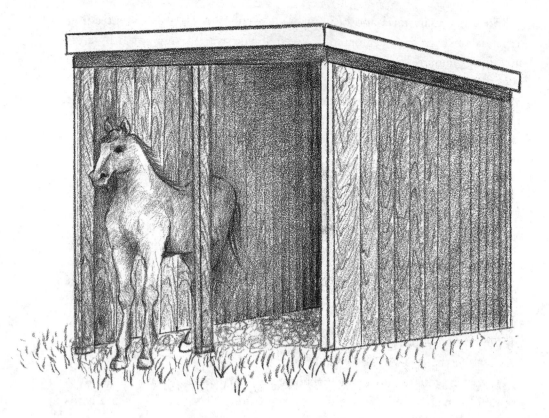

is wasted. You can reduce problems by picking up manure each day and making a compost pile in one corner. Most horses will learn to eliminate in that spot, so the job isn't as ominous as you'd expect.

What about pasture rotation? When done correctly, rotation serves several purposes: it allows for greater use of forage, and it helps reduce parasite transmission. Horses should begin to graze on pasture just before plant growth is complete. Remove the horses when forage height falls to three or four inches.

Keep the life cycle of equine parasites in mind when considering your pasture rotation plan. Rotation works only if the horses are kept off an area long enough to allow for death of most of the infective eggs and larvae, and the time that takes depends on the weather and on how well you clean up the pasture. If you are rotating your horses between two pastures every month or two, you may be exposing them to massive numbers of the parasites, since larvae will have had just enough time to hatch and climb the grass.

During the mild, wet days of spring and fall, the eggs mature rapidly, producing larvae within a week or two. Long periods of warm, dry weather or cold temperatures cause the eggs to delay maturation, but still survive. The eggs and hatching larvae can survive short freezes, too. These eggs hatch when adequate moisture and moderate temperatures resume. Extreme dry heat, long periods of freezing, or alternate freezes and thaws will kill parasite eggs and larvae.

Housing and
Diet

Spreading manure is another option. Destruction of eggs by spreading depends on extreme heat or cold. Even if you wait several months after spreading manure before you allow horses to graze, large numbers of infective eggs can still be present. Spreading manure during the mild, wet days of spring will only encourage hatching of the larvae. It is best not to spread manure on horse pasture.

Diet Essentials

Cover the Basics First

What do you feed your horse? Pasture or hay with some type of grain is the usual choice. All pastures and hays are not the same, though, and you may have mistaken ideas about feeding grain. When it comes to supplements, you'll be more confused than ever. Don't be swayed by flashy advertising.

How can you determine your horse's dietary needs? Basic guidelines are determined by the National Research Council (NRC). A special committee studies all available research on nutrition of horses. The result is a small booklet, "Nutrient Requirements of Horses," which gives dietary guidelines for all horses based on their weight, use, and age. (See appendix.)

You might be one of many who don't want to bother with reading such heavy material. Don't be concerned. If you own an adult horse that you ride for pleasure, you probably don't need to do an extensive feed analysis. However, you still need to put some thought into the type of feed your horse receives. First you must supply plenty of good-quality hay or pasture. Then you can decide whether your horse needs grain or a supplement.

What's best for your horse—hay, pasture, cubes, or pellets? No matter which form of roughage your horse receives, be sure that the diet you offer is of the best quality possible. Purchase feed from a reputable dealer. Your horse's feeding schedule and the type of feed you use should be consistent from day to day.

There are a few items in the "never-feed" category: lawn clippings, the remains of your brush-trimming job, and moldy hay or grain. Some people reason that lawn clippings are the same as pasture, so they offer a pile to their horse. The result could be severe indigestion, though, since the horse is not accustomed to that diet. Your lawn and garden could contain poisonous plants, too, so make a compost pile rather than offering the remains to your horse.

Whether your horse is on pasture or is fed hay, the best way to determine if he is getting enough to eat is to look at his condition. If your horse is healthy, not too fat and not too thin, then your feeding is probably right on target.

How can you tell if your horse is the correct weight? Each horse has a different build, so we can't recommend a certain weight according to height. Look at your horse from a short distance to judge his weight. Can you see the ribs? Does the croup look sharp and angular? If so, the horse is probably underweight.

Now look at your horse closely. Press your hand on its side and try to feel the ribs. If you cannot easily feel the ribs, your horse needs to go on a diet. Have your veterinarian take a look if you aren't sure.

Take care of parasite and tooth problems in the underweight horse. Next, be sure that the amount and quality of hay is adequate. Add grain to your horse's diet only after those items have been checked and the horse is still thin.

Pasture as Feed

Pasture is abundant in some parts of the country, and is a good choice for feeding some horses. Pasture quality varies depending on the type of grasses present, the number of horses grazing there, and on the time of year.

The number of horses per acre grazed varies with pasture quality. The best pasture might support one or two horses per acre, while fifty acres of dry range could barely support one horse. Horses with higher nutrient requirements because of exercise or growth might need extra hay or grain in addition to pasture. Other horses get fat on pasture and must be taken off for part of the day.

Many horses do fine on pasture during most of the year. They "unexpectedly" become thin in the fall or winter, when pasture grasses have matured to a point at which their nutrient levels are very low. Horses will continue to use their body reserves for a short time, but eventually will lose ground if their diets aren't supplemented.

Each part of the country will have a particular type of grass or legume that grows best. Because of differences in climate and soil conditions, recommendations for seeding, fertilization, and management of pasture will vary. Contact your county extension agent for specific help in this area.

Hay

If you aren't lucky enough to keep your horse on good pasture, the purchase of hay is a necessity. Several factors will influence your choice of hay.

Hay is cheaper by the ton, and buying large amounts ensures that your horse will receive a consistent diet. You must have storage space to keep it dry, though. If you live in a rural area, you might rent a large truck with your neighbors, and pick up and split a large load of hay between you.

Suburban horse owners will either use their stable's choice of hay, or will buy hay by the bale. You can still get some consistency in bales if you find a reputable hay lot and become a regular customer. Buy a new batch of hay before the old batch is entirely gone, then gradually mix the two. A sudden switch in hay could cause colic.

What Kind of Hay Should You Purchase? Basic types of hay include grass (such as timothy, bermuda, brome, orchard, or fescue hay), legume (such as alfalfa or red clover hay), or cereal (such as oat hay). Oat hay minus the cereal heads is just straw. If the cereal grains are left in, then oat hay is similar in nutritional content to grass hays.

Hay cubes or pellets are another choice. These have less dust and less waste than loose hay, an advantage for horses with chewing difficulties or respiratory disease.

The quality of pellets or cubes depends on the quality of the hay from which they're made, though, and you can't tell much by looking at the product. Another possible disadvantage is that horses without access to hay are deprived of their natural chewing tendencies, and may develop a wood-chewing vice.

What are the important ingredients of good hay? Horses need protein, carbohydrates (calories), vitamins and minerals in their diets. The adult horse requires 8 to 11 percent protein in its diet, which is easily supplied by most grass hays. Alfalfa hay has much higher protein levels, and is a good choice as part of the diet of most growing horses and brood mares.

Alfalfa hay is high in calcium and low in phosphorus; its ratio of calcium to phosphorus is about 6:1. Horses need a ratio of calcium to phosphorus between 1:1 and 3:1. For most horses, feeding alfalfa alone is not recommended.

Grass hay is lower in calories, vitamins, and some minerals than alfalfa hay. During periods of growth, nursing, or increased exercise, horses have specific vitamin and mineral needs, as well as higher caloric requirements. If these horses are fed grass hay, they'll need both grain and a vitamin-and-mineral supplement.

A combination of grass and alfalfa hay is ideal: it will provide the adult horse with a good balance of vitamins and minerals, and plenty of protein and calories to meet its needs.

No matter what type of hay you choose, it must be free of mold and weeds, feel soft and pliable, and look bright green. The leaves of alfalfa hay contain most of its nutrients, so be sure that the hay you choose is leafy, with fine stems.

Several different cuttings are typically made. The cutting with the highest nutritional value varies in different parts of the country. Slower growing periods (usually the first cutting) yield fewer stems and a higher nutritional content. However, first cuttings may have more weeds.

The cutting you buy is not as important as the stage of growth at which the hay is harvested. Hay that is cut at an early stage of maturity will have the most nutrients. Alfalfa should be cut at the bud stage (just before flowering), while grass hays should be cut just before they begin to show heads through the sheath.

Hay with high fiber or high moisture content should not be fed to horses. Hay that's baled with more than 15 to 20 percent moisture runs the risk of becoming moldy with storage, unless it has undergone acid treatment during baling. However, hay that is dried excessively will lose the leafy material, reducing its quality.

How Much and How Often Should You Feed Your Horse? Most of us are used to feeding a flake or two twice a day. But what's a flake? Different bales may form different sizes of flakes, and different people may grab a larger or smaller flake from a bale. The best thing to do is weigh a few of the typical flakes that you feed. Take your bathroom scale down to the barn and weigh yourself, plus and minus the flake, averaging out several flakes.

If different people are feeding your horse, you must all get together and show each other what you mean by a flake. That will avoid the mix-ups in communication that inevitably occur.

Once you've weighed your flake, calculate how much to feed your horse. Horses can eat up to 3 percent of their weight in feed per day. The "average" horse should consume 1 to 2 percent of its body weight in hay per day—that translates as ten to twenty pounds of hay for a thousand-pound horse. Divide that total amount into two or more feedings per day.

You'll feed the higher amount of hay to the horse that does not receive grain. If you feel that your horse has an unacceptable "hay belly," then cut back a little on the hay, and increase the grain.

Feeding hay pellets or cubes also requires careful measurement. Different pellets might be more or less compressed, so you cannot measure them by volume. A can full of small, tightly packed pellets contains more feed than the same can full of larger, softer cubes. Ask your feed store for specific recommendations on feeding the product that you buy.

How often should you feed hay? While a twice-daily feeding might be convenient for you, three or four meals are actually better for the horse. Most important is a consistent schedule every day, including weekends.

How should you feed your hay? From a rack or net, or on the ground? Each method has its advantages and disadvantages. Racks or nets should be high enough that the horse cannot catch a foot in one, yet not so high that hay and dust are falling in the horse's eyes and nose.

Feeding from the ground avoids those potential problems, but raises

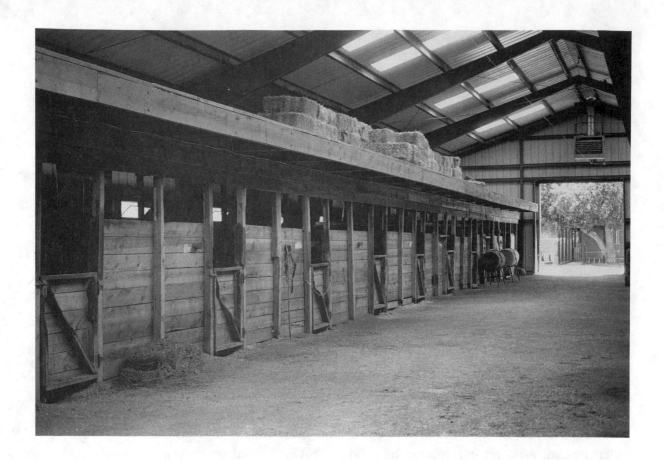

new ones. In sandy areas, horses fed from the ground risk dangerous buildup of sand in the intestine. Feeding from the ground could cause the horse to pick up parasite eggs. You can avoid these problems by providing a clean feeding area, such as a large rubber mat.

How Should You Store Your Hay? Carefully store your hay, cubes, or pellets. Your hay storage area can be as simple as a layer of well-spaced two-by-fours for a base and a well-secured tarp as a top.

In areas with much rain, you'll need better coverage. Use a stall in your barn or a separate shed. The worst place to store hay is in a barn loft above the horse's stalls. Even the best hay contains a great deal of dust, pollen, mold, and fungus spores. When hay is stored in a closed barn, the air your horses breathe can be very irritating to their lungs.

While your storage area must be dry, ventilation is important too. Allow some space between hay bales, because when slightly moist bales are tightly packed, heat can build up enough to cause a fire. Place a few well-spaced two-by-fours on a cement floor before stacking the bales to minimize condensation.

Cubes or pellets stored in a large bin can become moldy if stored

Easy Health Care
For Your Horse

improperly. Temperatures above 55°F, high humidity or moisture, and insect infestation can all promote mold growth.

How long can hay be stored? After several months, the hay will begin to loose its nutrients. Vitamins are gradually lost by oxidation and molds can continue to grow. The hay will dry out, becoming dustier and losing its leaves. If you must feed old hay, check it carefully for mold, and give your horse a vitamin supplement.

Hay has been fed for so long that few question its worth. Yet hay is not the horse's natural diet. One of the biggest differences between hay and pasture is the moisture content. Horses fed hay will drink much more water than those on pasture. Be sure that your horse has access to plenty of fresh water.

Blister Beetles

Blister beetles can contaminate hay and poison your horse when he eats. These beetles produce a chemical called cantharidin, which is very caustic. If even a few dead beetles are swallowed, they can irritate or destroy the lining of the intestinal tract. Symptoms of blister beetle poisoning range from mild colic to kidney failure, severe shock and death.

Blister beetle larvae emerge from the ground in the summer. The beetles tend to gather around blooming alfalfa hay in certain parts of the country. Some blister beetles feed on grasshoppers, so their numbers will increase during bad grasshopper years. The modern harvesting method of cutting and crimping in one operation prevents the beetles' escape, so they end up in the baled hay.

You can minimize the risk of blister beetle poisoning by buying good-quality alfalfa hay that has not yet bloomed. Early cuttings are less likely to be contaminated, since the beetles may not have emerged yet.

A Little Extra: Grain

Do you automatically dish out a can full of oats every day? What other grains are there to choose from? Is corn a "hotter" feed than oats? Does your horse actually need grain?

Chances are that you feed your horse based on what other people have fed theirs. That's a good way to start, but you need to open your mind to new ideas, both to improve your horse's health and to save money.

Does Your Horse Need Grain?

Why do you feed grain to your horse? Grain contains protein and carbohydrates. Since adult horses get plenty of protein from their hay, the only real nutrient grain provides to adult horses is carbohydrates, or calories. If your horse keeps weight on with good-quality hay, then you probably don't need to add grain to its diet.

Horses that are fed lower-quality hay, whether it be old or overmature, may not need the extra calories supplied by grain. It's more likely that those horses need a vitamin supplement. The lightly ridden pleasure horse that has trouble keeping on weight needs a good deworming and a dental exam before grain is automatically added to its diet.

Some horses have a big "hay belly," yet you can still easily feel their ribs. These horses probably aren't getting very good quality hay or pasture, so they must eat large amounts to meet their nutritional needs. After the deworming and dental exam, feed a little grain to see if that helps.

Your horse needs grain if he uses more energy than he can take in from hay or pasture alone. Pregnant mares, growing foals and yearlings, and horses under heavy exercise belong in this group. Use the previously mentioned guidelines to determine if your horse is underweight, and if so, add grain to the diet.

Grain can also be used as a protein source for growing horses (protein can also be provided with alfalfa hay or with such grain meals as soybean, cottonseed, or linseed meal). (See "Protein" section.)

Get a weight tape to help evaluate changes in your horse's diet. This measuring tape is placed around the horse's girth to provide a reading of the approximate weight of any horse with that girth measurement. The weight tape is not very accurate in determining the horse's exact weight, but you are more concerned with weight gain or loss. Any change in the tape measurement will reveal a change in weight, often before you notice anything obvious. Write down the measurement every week to evaluate your horse's progress.

How Much Grain Should You Feed?

How much grain should you feed? The answer is not in coffee can–fulls, because different grains have different weights. The weight of the grain determines its caloric content; this is called caloric density. For example, a one-pound coffee can full of corn weighs almost twice as much as the same can full of oats. If you feed them both by volume (a full one-pound coffee can), then you are feeding twice the amount of calories when you give the corn.

Take the time to weigh your coffee can with and without its load of grain so you really know how much you are feeding. One quart of oats weighs 1 pound, while a quart of barley weighs about 1.4 pounds and a quart of corn, 1.7 pounds.

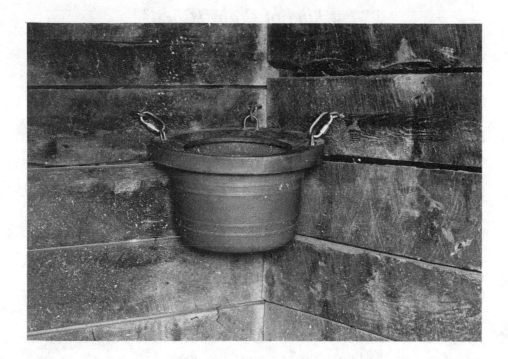

The amount you feed depends on how hard your horse is exercised and on its individual metabolism. Your horse can eat up to 3 percent of its body weight in feed per day. This will consist of ten to twenty pounds of hay, plus grain as needed. As a general rule, the weight of grain should never be more than the weight of hay consumed by your horse.

If your horse appears to need grain (as determined by its weight or exercise schedule), start with a general guideline of one-quarter to one-half pound of grain per one hundred pounds of horse. Feed about two to five pounds of grain each day, divided into two daily feedings. To be sure that horses kept together get their full daily portion of grain, you may have to separate them at feeding time.

If your horse has not received grain in the past, add it gradually to the diet. Slowly increase the amount of grain fed by one-half pound per day until you meet your goal. Changing the feed suddenly can expose your horse to the risk of colic, founder, or laminitis.

Watch your horse's weight over several weeks to help you determine whether you need to increase or decrease the amount of grain. Use your weight tape to help you notice and respond to small weight changes.

Take extra care if your horse is on an inconsistent exercise schedule. The classic muscle-soreness syndrome called "Monday morning disease" affects working horses that are rested over the weekend but continue to receive their regular amount of grain. The best way to feed is according to the amount of energy needed each day. Exercise should be consistent from day to day, even if you must hire someone to help you.

Housing and
Diet

What Kind of Grain Is Best?

Corn, oats, and barley are among the most popular grains. Oats are one of the most-used grains for horses, but are also among the most expensive. Oats are slightly higher in protein and lower in calories than corn. Since oats contain higher fiber and a lower level of calories by weight, they are safer to feed, since it is more difficult to give sufficient oats to cause digestive upset. Any grain can cause problems if it is overfed, however.

Barley is another good choice for grain. Some horses don't like the taste of barley as well as corn or oats, but it does well as part of a mix. Barley has about the same amount of protein as oats, and has a caloric density somewhere in between that of corn and oats.

While it is often the least expensive grain, many horse owners avoid feeding corn. Corn has an undeserved reputation as a "hot" feed, probably because its caloric density is so much higher than that of oats. People accustomed to feeding oats sometimes feed the same coffee can full of corn, and then wonder why their horses seem so full of energy. Remember, if you are feeding corn, you must use about half the volume you would feed of oats.

Corn will not cause a horse to founder more easily than will any other grain. The horse runs the risk of this disease if any grain is suddenly overfed. Perhaps because it is easily overfed by mistake, corn has an undeserved bad reputation for causing founder.

One problem with corn is that it is prone to mold. A dangerous fungus called *Fusarium* can grow on corn in a warm, moist environment. The *Fusarium* fungus produces a toxin called fumonisin, which causes "moldy corn poisoning" or leukoencephalomalacia, a deadly disease affecting the liver and the brain. Affected horses are weak and uncoordinated, and may become blind. There is no effective treatment.

Aflatoxins are produced by mold in corn and other feeds that are stored under high heat and humidity or corn that is stressed by drought during growth. High levels of aflatoxin are a big concern for cattle and pig farms, but they can also be a problem for horses. Weight loss and liver damage are common results of consuming aflatoxin. There are tests available that can measure the level of aflatoxin in corn.

You can avoid problems with corn by purchasing your grain from a reliable dealer and by taking a close look at the product yourself. Mold can form on the grain after it is purchased, too. Store your grain in a cool, dry area protected from the weather. Don't feed any suspicious-looking grain to your horse.

Easy Health Care
For Your Horse

Is Processed Grain Better?

You have many choices of grain, ranging from whole grains, to crimped or processed grains, to commercially prepared grain mixes that might have vitamins and minerals added. Your decision will be based on availability, cost, and your willingness to figure out your horse's ration. The budget-minded horse owner is better off buying whole grains, adding any needed supplements after careful calculation.

You have the option of purchasing cracked, crimped, or rolled grain instead of whole grain. Processed grain is slightly more digestible than whole grain. Horses with dental problems and older horses will benefit from receiving processed grain. Because its outer hull is cracked or crimped, processed grain is more susceptible to deterioration and mold, and cannot be stored for as long as whole grain.

Is processed grain a better buy? Processing can increase the availability of nutrients in corn by 7 to 9 percent and in oats by 2 to 5 percent. If processed corn costs over 9 percent more than unprocessed corn, or processed oats over 5 percent more than unprocessed, then the unprocessed grain is actually the better buy.

Another choice is the convenient bags of commercial grain mixes with vitamins and minerals added. These products appear to be a good buy, since the supplement is already there in theoretically correct amounts. (Remember, don't feed an additional vitamin or mineral supplement if you are already feeding supplemented grain). The precise level of nutrients in the adult pleasure horse's diet isn't critical, and premixed feeds are quite convenient. If your horse is receiving good-quality hay, though, you may not need those extras. Your money might be better spent purchasing grain alone.

Even though they are labeled for certain groups of horses (growth, exercise, and brood mares), commercial grain mixes are made for the average horse of that type. They are not prepared with your specific type and quality of hay in mind. Your horse might receive too much of some nutrients and not enough of others. If you own a brood mare or growing horse, devote the extra time and effort to evaluating its ration. Your vet probably has a copy of the National Research Council (NRC) book and can help you design a balanced diet (see appendix).

So, How Much Hay and Grain Should I Feed?

All right, you've read the whole chapter up to here and you're still wondering why someone doesn't just say: "Feed x pounds of hay and x pounds of oats." Although that would seem an easy solution, it would

Housing and
Diet

be a disservice to you and your horse in the long run. Every horse has a different exercise schedule, different needs, and a different quality of feed.

Reread the above sections until you feel comfortable with the questions how, why, and when you should make changes in your horse's diet. Here's a general idea of where to start your feeding schedule.

The total amount of feed should equal 1 to 3 percent of the horse's body weight, or ten to thirty pounds of feed daily for a one thousand-pound horse (weigh your horse and adjust the following figures appropriately). If you feed only hay, offer twenty pounds per day; weight it to see how many flakes that is.

If your horse is exercised moderately, you probably need to add grain to its diet; lower the amount of hay to about fifteen pounds, and feed two to five pounds of grain (not two to five one-pound coffee-canfuls; *two to five pounds of grain*). For heavy exercise, feed eight to ten pounds of hay and five to eight pounds of grain. Racehorses and top athletes consume even more grain than that.

Decide the amount you are going to feed and stick with that amount for several weeks. Measure your horse with a weight tape once a week to watch his progress. Increase or decrease grain by about a half-pound at a time, once again feeding the same amount for several weeks to find the level of feed at which your horse maintains body weight.

Nutritional Supplements

Everyone shares that exasperated feeling you get when you walk into a feed store. Shelves are piled high with hundreds of products, all claiming to make your horse healthier, happier, or a better athlete; they'll make him grow bigger and stronger than the rest, perk up, or calm down; his hooves will be transformed from dry and flaky to shiny and strong, and his coat will bloom as never before. If your horse was doing just fine, there are products to make him even better.

There is no simple way to choose the right supplement for your horse. The area of the country where you live and the type of hay and grain you feed have a profound effect on your horse's nutrient intake. Deciding on the best supplement will require a little work on your part, but your horse is surely worth the effort. Before you go out and buy a vitamin supplement, check the feed your horse is getting now. Perhaps the feed already meets your horse's requirements.

The horse requires several basic nutrients: water, protein, energy, vitamins, and minerals. If you look up the requirements for an adult horse on a moderate exercise schedule, you'll find that you're well within safe limits—he has all of his needs met with good quality pasture or grass–alfalfa hay, fresh water, and a trace-mineral salt block.

Most adult pleasure horses do just fine on a diet of hay. When your horse works harder, he eats more, and more nutrients (protein, vitamins, and minerals) are taken in. You don't need to add any supplements because of increased exercise if your horse has plenty of good-quality hay. Feed grain as needed to meet the energy (calorie) demands of an increased exercise schedule.

Vitamin or mineral excess can harm your horse, so beware of supplementing when it's not needed. For example, selenium is deficient in many areas, and it has become popular to supplement this mineral. However, in other areas of the country selenium levels are dangerously high. Supplementing in these cases will cause signs of selenium toxicity, including brittle hooves, poor coat, blindness, and incoordination.

You must keep your own goals in mind. Much of the material you read about dietary recommendations doesn't even apply to your horse. Get together with your veterinarian to discuss any changes you want to make.

What Supplement Does Your Horse Need?

What horses need a nutritional supplement? First, any horse fed brown or old hay is not getting proper nutrition. Also, athletes, growing horses, and sick horses all might need a supplement. Take care of the basics first, though. A horse with sharp teeth or worms won't look too sprightly, and a supplement won't change that.

As a general rule, get a supplement that provides no more than 100 percent of your horse's daily requirements with each dose, and which contains a balance of vitamins and minerals. If you are already feeding a supplemented grain mix, then don't add a vitamin or mineral supplement to your horse's diet, since you could overdose some nutrients. More is not better.

Your horse's health depends not only on how much of each nutrient is in the diet, but also on the precise balance and ratios of each nutrient to the others. Never supplement just one vitamin or mineral unless you have had your horse's ration analyzed.

The best way to tell if your horse has a deficiency or excess of a particular nutrient is to have your hay analyzed. If you buy in small quantities, you can instead get a general idea of the nutrient content of hay and grain from nutritional tables such as those in the NRC's book (see appendix).

Feed analysis will give you an estimate of your horse's overall nutritional level and levels of some specific nutrients, but doesn't consider any of the interactions between nutrients that occur after eating. For example, a large amount of copper could interfere with selenium absorption, even if the level of selenium by itself is adequate.

Blood tests theoretically tell you which nutrients the horse has absorbed, but are not always an accurate measure. Blood testing seems to work well enough for selenium and gives some sign of copper status, but is not accurate for other nutrients. For example, the horse's body places high priority on proper blood calcium levels. Calcium is drawn from the bone to keep the blood levels in the normal range when the amount ingested is low.

Hair analysis is used to check for toxic levels of certain minerals, such as selenium or zinc. Dirt on the hair can totally alter the results, and the levels measured will reflect the horse's nutrient intake at the time the hair grew out—possibly months earlier. Hair does not always collect nutrients in the same amounts in which they are ingested, and the levels may vary with hair color.

You can have a water analysis done when inexplicable problems cannot be traced to the feed. Water may be contaminated with high levels of zinc, selenium, or nitrates.

Let's take a look at the ingredients of various supplements and the functions they perform for the horse. Although each nutrient is discussed separately, it's not a good idea to add just one or another to your horse's feed without careful analysis, because you can throw off his entire nutrient balance.

There are maximum as well as minimum levels for optimal nutrition, as well as specific ratios that must be met. Each nutrient depends on the others for optimal action. (For information on laxatives, natural supplements, and miscellaneous additives, see chapter 10, "Alternative Medicine and Therapy".)

Minerals

Should you supplement minerals in your horse's diet? In most cases, feeding good-quality hay with free access to a trace-mineral salt block will provide your horse with adequate levels. Since the success of a block depends on the horse taking in the correct amounts, some people prefer to give a premeasured amount of a loose salt mix instead.

Don't supply both a plain salt block and a trace-mineral block. Your horse can't tell how much of each he should take in. Just supply one block that's made for horses and contains both salt and trace minerals. If you are sure that you live in (and use hay from) a selenium-deficient area, then get a block that contains extra selenium.

Growing horses, nursing mares, and athletic horses that sweat a great deal (endurance horses, for example) might need additional minerals or a specially formulated supplement (see following sections).

Macro minerals include calcium, phosphorus, potassium, and magnesium. Most adult horses will get an adequate amount of these minerals with good-quality hay or pasture.

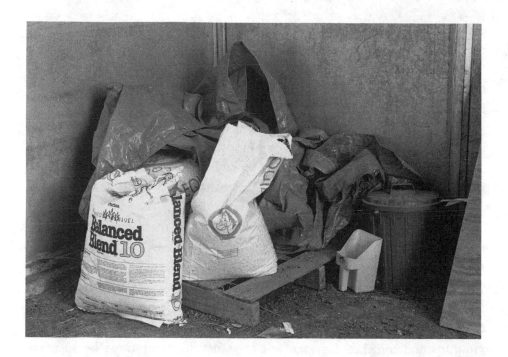

Calcium and phosphorus are necessary for normal bone development, and a proper ratio between them is essential for growing horses and brood mares. Alfalfa hay is high in calcium and low in phosphorus, while grass hay is low in both, and grain is high in phosphorus. Beware of any supplement that doesn't consider hay type in its instructions. To be safer yet, only add these minerals after you know how much of each your horse's diet requires.

Sodium chloride, or salt, is essential in maintaining the body's water balance. Potassium is necessary for many bodily functions, including muscle action. Hay naturally contains potassium. Magnesium interacts with calcium and phosphorus in bone development. Most horses get all the magnesium they need from their hay.

Trace Minerals include selenium, copper, zinc, iron, iodine, cobalt, and manganese. These minerals are found in hay, molasses, and in trace-mineral salt blocks. In special cases, supplements might be needed.

Selenium acts with vitamin E to stabilize cell membranes. Deficiencies result in muscle problems, but not all muscle problems improve with supplementation of this mineral. The amount of selenium in your horse's hay or pasture varies widely with the region of the country. In some areas, excess selenium leads to problems of toxicity. In other areas a selenium deficiency exists. If you live in a selenium-deficient area, it's worthwhile to have your hay analyzed so you'll know how much you need to supplement.

Copper is necessary for normal blood, skin, hair, and bone development. Copper has complex interactions with other minerals. For example,

Housing and
Diet

copper ties up selenium and competes with zinc. Recent evidence shows that some hay may be low in the copper levels needed for growing horses.

Many of the body's enzymes contain zinc, which is also necessary for normal skin. High levels of zinc may lead to copper deficiency and problems in bone development.

Iron is a normal part of blood and several body proteins. Although iron is present in many "blood buildups," low iron is not a common cause of anemia in horses. Anemic horses won't usually improve with iron supplementation. A better idea is to have the cause of the anemia diagnosed and then treat the problem accordingly.

Iodine is a part of the thyroid hormones. An increase or decrease of iodine can cause goiter, an enlargement of the thyroid gland. Iodine toxicity has been caused by some products containing kelp (seaweed); check the label carefully for iodine levels. Cobalt is necessary for vitamin B_{12} production. A deficiency of either cobalt or B_{12} has not been seen in horses. Manganese is essential for bone and cartilage formation. All the vitamins and minerals necessary for bone development must be supplied together in the correct amounts and proportions.

Vitamins

Vitamins are either fat-soluble (A, D, E, and K) or water-soluble (B complex and C). Fat-soluble vitamins can be stored in your horse's body for long periods. Water-soluble vitamins are excreted in the urine, so they need to be replenished each day.

Water-Soluble Vitamins are found in abundance in good hay. Horses that are ill or under extreme stress, such as athletes or show horses, may need a supplement.

Vitamin C plays a role in wound healing; it may be fed to horses in the form of ascorbyl palmitate or ascorbic acid. Two relatives of vitamin C, hesperidin complex and lemon bioflavonoids, are relatively new ingredients in many supplements.

The vitamin B complex includes thiamine (B_1), riboflavin (B_2), pantothenic acid (B_3), pyridoxine (B_6), folic acid (B_{10}), cyanocobalamin (B_{12}), choline, inositol, niacin, biotin, and PABA. What is sometimes referred to as vitamin B_{15} is not a vitamin at all (see chapter 10, *Alternative Medicine and Therapy*). Biotin is needed for normal skin, hair, and hoof growth. B_1, B_3, and B_6 are needed for normal nervous system function. B_6, B_{12}, and folic acid are used by red blood cells.

Fat-Soluble Vitamins are stored in the body for many months after ingestion, so they may reach toxic levels when overfed. Poor-quality hay or hay that has been stored a long time may be low in vitamins A and E.

Vitamin A or its precursor, beta carotene, are needed for the eyes, skin, and mucus membranes. There is plenty of beta carotene in any green feed, but it will be low in brown or old hay.

Vitamin D is produced naturally by the interaction of the sun on your horse's skin; a couple of hours of sunlight daily are all that is necessary. Sun-cured hay also contains vitamin D. This vitamin interacts with calcium and phosphorus in the normal formation of bone.

Vitamin E plays a role in healing, reproduction, in muscular function and in the nervous system. Side effects of high levels of vitamin E have not been reported, distinguishing it from the other fat-soluble vitamins.

Vitamin K is necessary for normal blood clotting. Fortunately, vitamin K is made in adequate amounts by the bacteria in your horse's gut, and a deficiency is practically unheard of. Vitamin K injections have caused toxic reactions in horses.

Protein and Amino Acids

Protein is made up of amino acids. Adult horses have low protein requirements, which are easily met with good hay or pasture. Horses fed more protein than they need will convert it into energy or body fat, not extra muscle. Those extra calories an be provided more effectively in other ways. A high-protein diet will also make your horse urinate more, making his kidneys work harder and increasing your stall-cleaning time.

Nursing mares and growing foals need extra protein. Both the amount and the quality of protein are important. Good alfalfa hay has a high level of protein. Lysine is an essential amino acid found in alfalfa hay and soybean meal; it is low in many other feeds.

Other plant protein sources include soybean, cottonseed, or linseed meal. Of these, soybean meal is the best choice, since it contains lysine. Linseed meal was used in the past because it added a "bloom" to a horse's coat; modern production of linseed meal takes out the oil, though, so that benefit no longer exists. Animal-source protein supplements include fish meals and dairy products.

Amino acids, including tyrosine, tryptophan, phenylalanine, aspartic acid and histidine, are a common ingredient of many supplements that are made for specific problems. Methionine helps horses with founder. Other amino acids are found in special formulas designed to perk up, calm down, or relieve pain in your horse.

Supplement Labels

Even the most experienced horse owners are often baffled at the sight of a supplement label. Ask them what the ingredients mean, what they do, and whether the amounts correspond to their horse's daily requirements, and they're often at a loss for an answer.

You're probably a smart buyer interested in learning more about any product before you give it to your horse. You can learn why some of the things you hear should be ignored, and the glimmer of truth behind others.

How are you supposed to read those labels, anyway? When you shop for a supplement, remember these important tips.

Be wary of new (but "essential") nutrients; just because an ingredient is on the label doesn't mean it's needed by your horse.

Don't simply pick the product with the most ingredients in the highest amounts.

Ignore your tendency to think that a little of everything covers all the bases.

"Natural" products or those made from herbs or seaweed aren't always better.

Do your horse a favor and don't just take something off the shelf because it looks good. Although labels for horse vitamins don't list the Recommended Daily Allowances as your own do, you can get this information from the NRC's "Nutrient Requirements for Horses" (See appendix). Compare your horse's feed with his nutrient requirements, then compare the nutrients he lacks with the product label to see if it's appropriate for him. That way, you'll avoid paying for extra nutrients your horse doesn't need, and you won't be swayed by manufacturer's claims or tantalizing labels.

Unfortunately, it is not that simple. When you take a look at several different labels you'll be amazed at all the different ways a nutrient can be listed. IUs (International Units) per pound, milligrams per ounce, or percentages can be seen on the same label. The same ingredient may be listed under different names, giving you a mistaken impression (for example, beta carotene and vitamin A; or ascorbic acid, vitamin C, and ascorbyl palmitate). You might have to do a little math to figure out exactly how much of each nutrient is actually in a daily dose of some supplements.

First, look to see if the amounts are listed per container or per daily dose. If they are listed per container, you will have to divide the amount listed by the number of doses. Once you've converted each nutrient into its daily amount, you need to change the units to those used in the NRC's book. Some useful conversion factors:

1 kg	= 2.2 lb.	8 oz.	= 1 cup	1 cc	= 1 ml
1 oz.	= 28.35 g	1 g	= 1000 mg	1 mg	= 1000 mcg
1 IU	= 1 USP unit	1 oz.	= 30 ml	1 mg	= 64.8 grains
1 tbsp.	= 3 tsp.	g/kg × 0.1 = %		1 tsp.	= 5 g or 5 ml

mg beta carotene × 400 = IU vitamin A

How much is enough? A supplement providing more than 100 percent of your horse's daily requirements is a waste of your money, and may be harmful. Ideally, you'll be providing just what is missing from his hay and grain.

Call or write the company—most are happy to talk with you and answer your questions. Ask for their product literature and experimental data, then analyze the information with the help of your veterinarian.

Special Claims

Many products make special claims, such as "chelated minerals," "natural" or "water-soluble vitamin A." What do these statements actually mean?

Chelated minerals are attached to another substance to increase their absorption. Products containing chelated minerals are more expensive. If a product doubles a mineral's absorption by chelation but its cost is more than double, then the nonchelated product may be the best buy.

Older horses with reduced ability to digest and absorb nutrients may benefit from chelated minerals. Chelated minerals may also be useful when high levels of one mineral exist in the diet; chelation might then help prevent antagonism that would prevent absorption of other nutrients. High copper levels, for example, interfere with zinc absorption.

Water soluble forms of vitamins A, D, and E are sometimes advertised. These fat-soluble vitamins are stored in the body, and may produce toxic effects if overdosed over time (in any form). "Water soluble" may mean emulsified. "Water soluble" vitamin A usually means beta carotene. Don't be mislead—while absorption may improve, these products aren't any safer than the others when it comes to overdosage.

Natural products sound appealing. Unfortunately, use of the word *natural* is not regulated on equine feeds and supplements, so any company can use the term on a label. (See chapter 10 for more on what "natural" means.)

Supplements for
the Growing Horse

Young horses, up to two years old, have higher protein and energy requirements than adults, and adequate vitamin and mineral levels are even more important. While an adult might get by with a minor nutrient deficiency, the same diet in a young horse results in growth deformities.

The quality of protein is important, too. Amino acids, the building blocks of protein, should be present in the proper amounts. The amino acid lysine is most often deficient in the foal's ration. Alfalfa hay and soybean meal contain lysine, but it is low in many other feeds.

Mineral imbalances may predispose the growing horse to bone disease. Although restricting protein and carbohydrates will slow growth and avoid problems, balancing the mineral levels might also be necessary. A custom-made supplement is a better idea than free-choice minerals for the foal.

Analyze the ration with your vet's help. Most often, you'll need to adjust the calcium and phosphorus levels or their ratio to each other. Young horses fed alfalfa hay will tend toward calcium excess and phosphorus deficiency, while those fed grass hay might have the opposite problem, with a calcium deficiency.

Supplements for the Athlete

Dietary supplements for athletic horses are designed to meet a variety of needs. The athlete may be a racehorse, endurance horse, hardworking show horse, or rodeo competitor.

The athletic horse's main deficiency is likely to be caloric; add grain as needed (use your weight tape to monitor your horse's progress). Although their protein requirements are slightly higher, these horses don't need any extra protein in their diets. When you increase the feed to provide extra calories, you are automatically providing more of each of the nutrients, including protein, in the ration.

Fat is added to the diet of many horses to meet their increased caloric needs. Sometimes these horses just can't consume enough grain, and vegetable oil provides more calories with less bulk. (See chapter 10 for more information.) Oil is also used for "glycogen loading" before endurance races, but whether this provides any observable advantage is controversial.

"Thumps," or synchronous diaphragmatic flutter, occurs in some horses during or after exercise. Contractions of the diaphragm are seen as a twitching in the flank area with every heartbeat. Thumps are due to changes in blood calcium and other electrolytes. Sometimes a change in the horse's ration can help prevent the problem. (See "Exercise-Associated Problems" in chapter 8.)

Electrolytes (calcium, sodium, potassium, and other salts) are given to athletes to replace those lost in sweat. Electrolytes work best when given after the losses have occurred, rather than continuously in the feed. Consult your veterinarian for specific recommendations about electrolytes, since the type of exercise your horse does determines which electrolytes are needed.

Sodium chloride (table salt), potassium chloride (salt substitute), and calcium are among the electrolytes given. One commonly used mixture is half salt substitute (the kind that is half sodium chloride and half potassium chloride) and half table salt. Give the electrolytes just before, during, and after competition.

Salt, sodium bicarbonate, selenium, and other supplements may be used for horses with muscle problems. Be sure to have your veterinarian examine any horse with a continual muscle problem, though, since there are many causes and each is treated differently.

A recent study showed that blood levels of thiamine and folic acid, two B vitamins, may be low in some racehorses. Another study showed that stressed horses had a mild depletion of vitamin C. The recommended daily requirement for vitamin E has been raised. Research on the nutrition of stressed athletic horses continues, so keep your ears open for news. (See chapter 10 for more on blood buildups, bleeding remedies, special nutrients, and jugs.)

The Older Horse

Aged horses have a decreased ability to store vitamins and minerals. They may have tooth problems that result in decreased intake or improper chewing of food, and they might have decreased organ function. But with good health care, we're seeing horses live well into their thirties.

Some older horses need a change from hay to an easily chewable feed. Offer pellets or a gruel. A balanced vitamin–mineral supplement is a good idea for the aged horse.

Ask your vet about blood chemistry tests to check your older horse's liver and kidney function. If problems exist, a change in the type of feed may be helpful.

Health Problems and the Diet

Dietary changes or supplements can help certain health problems.

Poor hoof growth, and flaky, dry, or cracked hooves can have several causes. Analyze your ration first. Deficiencies in protein, calcium, and many different vitamins and minerals can cause hoof problems. Several supplements might improve hoof growth, strength, and resiliency. Whether your horse will respond to any of these depends on the cause of his problem, but it's worth a try. Biotin, a B vitamin, improves hoof quality in many cases. Methionine, an amino acid, helps horses with chronic founder. Often these substances are combined with others in hoof-improver products.

The sick horse, no matter what his illness, has an increased need for nutrients, since his body uses them up faster. In addition, illness often dulls the appetite, so the horse has even greater deficiencies. The sick horse needs extra vitamins B and C. B vitamins have the additional advantage of stimulating appetite.

Horses with diarrhea and other gastrointestinal problems also have extra nutrient requirements—they are losing nutrients faster than they're taking them in. Both the fat-soluble and water-soluble vitamins will be in short supply. In some cases, "probiotics" (supplements containing live bacteria) may help the horse reestablish its normal gut organisms.

Liver, kidney, or heart problems, all long-term diseases, require special dietary considerations. Your veterinarian can help you formulate a special diet for a variety of disease conditions.

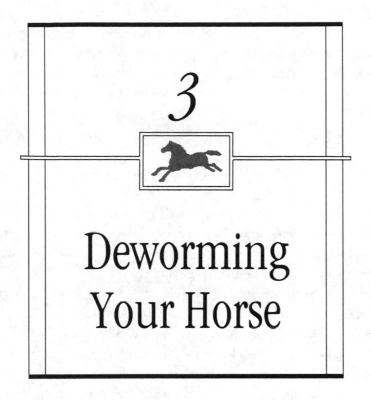

3

Deworming Your Horse

Internal Parasites

Your horse's colic episode came as a complete surprise. After all, the horse looked great and was performing well. The vet's diagnosis of a parasite problem was even more unexpected. You had been using paste dewormers regularly, changing products each time. What could have gone wrong?

Signs of parasite damage can vary from none at all to rough coat, pot belly, weight loss, and colic. Your horse may appear to be fine, yet internal damage continues until an episode of colic ensues. Worms and their eggs are everywhere, and can survive for long periods. Your horse is guaranteed to be exposed. With all the controversy surrounding deworming programs and the effectiveness of different dewormers, how do you decide which program and which products are best for your situation?

First, become familiar with the different parasites that could affect your horse. Then get to know the types of dewormers available and how and when to use them. That way, you can avoid using products that aren't effective and you'll be sure that your rotational program is really doing its job.

Bots

The little yellowish dots on your horse's lips and front legs appear harmless at first, but several months from now those botfly eggs will have developed into larvae in your horse's stomach. Your horse is sure to be infested with bots unless your area is entirely free of flies.

Bots are the larvae of the *Gasterophilus* fly. Since these flies can't live through the cold months of winter, they have developed a unique method of ensuring the survival of future generations. The small, yellowish flies (which look a little like bees) live only for a week or so as adults, spending most of their lives as immature bots in the horse's stomach.

Botflies start laying their eggs in the spring and summer, with a peak egg-laying period in the fall. The season can extend almost year-round in warmer climates. The eggs hatch when the horse rubs or licks his legs with his lips and tongue. Tiny immature larvae latch onto the horse's mouth and burrow into the tissues. A large infestation may cause tenderness and ulcers throughout your horse's mouth.

The larvae spend a month or two maturing in the tongue before they emerge and are swallowed. Over the next several weeks, they grow and develop into stomach bots.

Bots create deep pits in the stomach wall. Severe cases may cause perforation of the stomach or blockage of its outflow into the small intestine. Bots can live attached to the stomach wall for up to a year before they finally release their hold and are expelled in the manure. They spend another month or two on the ground and then hatch into adult botflies.

There is no simple way to diagnose bot infestations. You can assume that horses with eggs on their legs and face are infested with bots.

A bot treatment has traditionally been recommended after the first killing frost each year, when all adult flies have died. While this advice is well taken, you are leaving your horses open to infestation the rest of the year if you don't treat more often.

Botflies begin to deposit their eggs in early spring. If you don't use a

Easy Health Care
For Your Horse

boticide (bot treatment) until November, you're leaving bots in your horse's stomach all summer long. Treatments in spring, summer, and fall are a good idea. The organophosphates and ivermectin kill both bots at the tongue-migrating stage and bots in the stomach.

Fly control is as important as regular bot treatments. (See chapter 6 for details.) Regular manure cleanup will keep any hatching botflies away from your horse. Remember to shave the eggs off your horse's hair after your last bot treatment in the fall.

Several products provide feed-through fly control. These products contain low levels of organophosphates, which remove the bots from the horse's stomach. The drug persists in manure, killing the larvae of flies that lay eggs in compost.

The low levels of drug in feed-through products may not be enough to remove all the bots from your horse. If you're using a feed-through product regularly, be aware that you may overdose your horse by deworming him with an organophosphate (trichlorfon or dichlorvos) paste or tube product (See "Deworming Products," below.) Also, be sure you're environmentally responsible in the disposal of manure that contains chemicals.

Ascarids (Roundworms)

While older horses are plagued with strongyles, the young horse from birth to two years is also affected by roundworms (ascarids, or *Parascaris equorum*). Even though this parasite is killed by many dewormers, it remains a threat and a problem.

Ascarid eggs are almost indestructible. The hard little shell surrounding an immature larva withstands freezing and heat, extreme wet and desiccating dryness. The egg can live for years if need be, waiting for an opportunity to infect another foal. Many disinfectants don't affect these eggs at all.

Adult ascarids are extremely prolific. An infected horse may pass millions of eggs in its manure each day. These sticky eggs are easily transported on your feet or on shovels and other barn equipment. Even a farm with a modern deworming program and impeccable hygiene can have problems with roundworm infestation.

We typically think of intestinal damage from worms, but ascarids migrate through many body tissues. Once the eggs are ingested, small larvae hatch out into the foal's intestine, then migrate through the liver and lungs. Ascarids are a frequent cause of cough in the foal. The larvae are coughed up and swallowed, returning to the foal's intestine, where they grow to adult worms.

The time span from the foal's first infection to the time eggs are passed

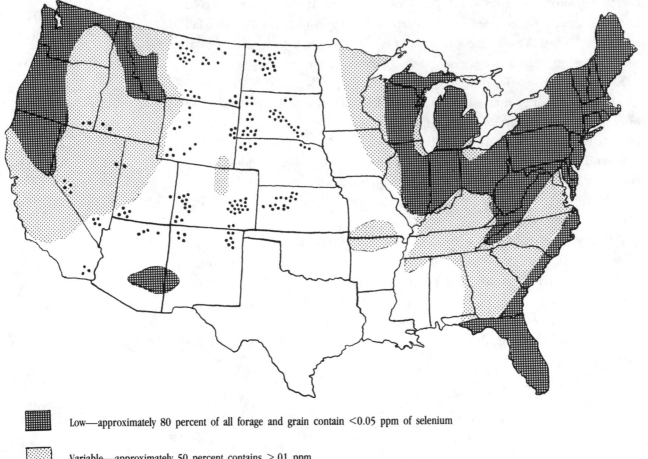

in its manure is eighty days or more. Foals younger than three months may have negative fecal egg counts and still be heavily infested from the day they are born.

The first step in an effective control program is removing the source of infestation. While you'll never get rid of all the eggs, you can reduce their numbers considerably. Daily removal of manure is essential. Use a product such as Lysol, a phenol-based disinfectant, to scrub down stalls. Manure control in the pasture is as important as in the barn.

Start your deworming program without waiting for large numbers of eggs to appear in your horse's manure. By then, contamination of the premises with millions more eggs has already happened. No matter what product you use, your horse is reinfested almost immediately, so you must keep with the program.

Most dewormers are effective against ascarids, including piperazine, pyrantel, the benzimidazoles (except thiabendazole) and ivermectin.

Easy Health Care
For Your Horse

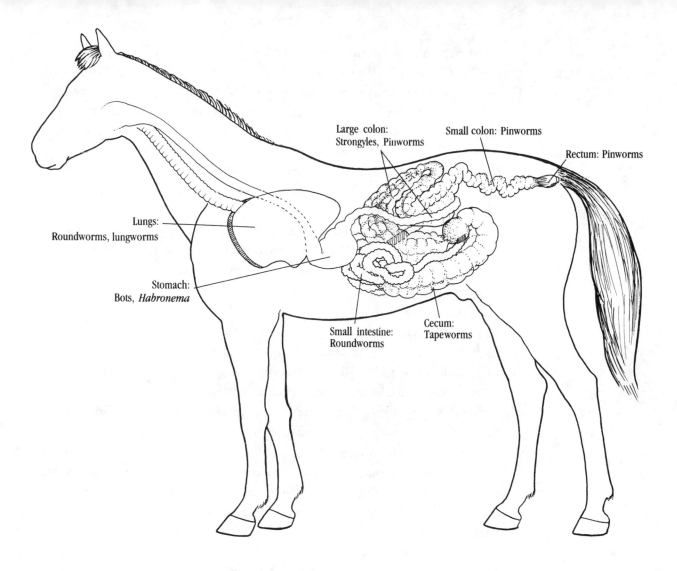

Large colon:
Strongyles, Pinworms

Small colon: Pinworms

Rectum: Pinworms

Lungs:
Roundworms, lungworms

Stomach:
Bots, *Habronema*

Small intestine:
Roundworms

Cecum:
Tapeworms

Older horses seldom have a problem with ascarids. As the horse matures, it gradually builds up an immunity to these worms. The larvae are destroyed as they migrate through the liver and lungs.

Strongyles (Bloodworms)

Larvae of the strongyle family are one of the most devastating parasites that can affect your horse. The three types of large strongyles, *Strongylus vulgaris*, *Strongylus edentatus*, and *Strongylus equinus*, each create a different problem. After arriving in the intestine, the larvae begin a migratory stage. It's often a year or more after the eggs first enter the horse's body that the adult finally develops. Adult large strongyles may cause diarrhea and anemia, but the immature larvae create much more damage.

S. edentatus migrates through the liver, and *S. equinus* travels through the abdominal wall, abdominal cavity, and pancreas. *S. vulgaris* is the most damaging species; its larvae migrate into the arteries supplying the

53

Deworming
Your Horse

intestine, causing inflammation, thickening, and disruption of the blood supply to the gut. The duration and severity of infestation determines whether damage caused by large strongyles is permanent or reversible.

Poor blood supply leads to inadequate function of the intestine, which makes the horse much more susceptible to colic. Weakening of the blood vessel walls can result in an aneurysm, an enlarged area that may suddenly rupture and cause the horse to bleed to death. Since damage is done long before the adults ever lay eggs, a negative fecal (manure) egg count does not prove absence of the worms.

Larvae return to the intestine, mature, and produce eggs that are passed in the horse's manure. The eggs and infective larvae that develop from them can survive for a long time in your pasture before being picked up by a grazing horse.

If you use a deworming product that kills only the adult stages of strongyles, maturing larvae will continually emerge from your horse's tissues into his gut, creating constant problems. Ivermectin, fenbendazole, and oxfendazole kill the migrating stages; ask your veterinarian for other suggestions, since recommendations change frequently.

Small strongyles (*Cyathostomes*) also live in the large intestine. Small strongyle larvae may quickly mature to adults, or they can penetrate the intestinal wall, forming cysts or nodules. The cysts may mature in as little as two months. At other times, usually over the winter, larvae persist in the nodules for longer periods. Wintertime manure samples may be entirely devoid of worm eggs even though the horse is infested with parasites.

Small strongyles mature and lay eggs in the spring and summer. Maturing larvae can emerge from the cysts in a sudden migration that causes severe damage and an intense inflammatory reaction, a common cause of springtime colic.

Small strongyles have developed resistance to many different deworming chemicals over the past several decades. Follow your veterinarian's advice and use a product that overcomes any drug-resistance problems in your area.

Repeat your dewormings every two months, since a small strongyle egg may be ingested and mature to an egg-laying adult after only six weeks. Your goal is to prevent any more eggs from being spread.

Control of small strongyles must also include periodic use of a drug that is effective against the encysted larvae. Treatment is especially important during the winter to prevent your horse from becoming ill in the spring when the encysted stages emerge.

Few dewormers are effective against the tissue stages of these parasites. Larvae may be killed by ivermectin or by using a larger dose of one of the benzimidazoles over several days' time. This is an off-label use and should be done only by a veterinarian. Horses having recurring colic problems due to strongyle migration may need special treatment.

Pinworms

Pinworms (*Oxyuris equi*) are one cause of the "itchy-tail syndrome." The adult pinworm lives in the large intestine, but doesn't cause much disturbance there. Pinworms deposit their eggs around the anus, causing irritation, itching, tail-rubbing, and hair loss.

Eggs can fall to the ground or are deposited wherever the horse rubs its rear end. Horses are reinfected with pinworms when they ingest larvae that hatch from eggs several days later.

Your veterinarian will do a "scotch-tape prep" to diagnose pinworms, since there are other causes of tail-rubbing (see chapter 6). A piece of scotch tape is pressed around the horse's anus, then pressed onto a microscope slide so the tiny pinworm eggs can be examined.

Pinworms are easily treated with many dewormers, including the benzimidazoles, ivermectin, and the organophosphates.

Tapeworms

Anaplocephala perfoliata and *Anaplocephala magna*, the equine tapeworms, are less commonly diagnosed than the other parasites. Tapeworms have an interesting life cycle, which involves a stage inside a mite. The mite eats the worm egg in the manure, the horse eats the mite, and the immature tapeworm then emerges and develops into an adult.

Adult tapeworms live in and near the horse's cecum, a large dead-end extension between the small and large intestine. Large numbers of tapeworms may cause blockage of the opening into the cecum, ulcers, or even rupture of the intestine.

Tapeworms can be difficult to diagnose. A standard fecal egg count may or may not reveal the eggs, and the worms are seldom seen in the manure. Many of the dewormers in use today, including ivermectin, are not effective against tapeworms. Your veterinarian will help you choose the medication to eradicate this parasite.

Other Parasites

There are many other worms that infest horses, but they probably won't be a problem for you.

Strongyloides (thread worm) is a small worm that can cause diarrhea in foals. The immature larvae of this parasite can pass through the mare's milk to the foal. Owners of pregnant mares should deworm the mare with ivermectin the day that she gives birth to remove any larvae in her mammary gland. Several different dewormers will kill the worms in the foal.

Habronema larvae live in the stomach wall, where they form tumorlike growths. These worms are also the cause of summer sores on the horse's outer body (see chapter 6). While the stomach parasite is difficult to diagnose, it is killed by ivermectin, so you are probably eliminating any problem by using that drug in your program.

Dictyocaulus is a lung worm of horses and donkeys. Infection with lung worms will cause a chronic cough. Immature lung worm larvae are coughed up and swallowed, so they may be seen by microscopic examination of your horse's manure. Ivermectin kills these parasites.

Fasciola hepatica, the liver fluke, is a parasite of cattle and sheep that occasionally infests the horse. Signs include weight loss, colic, and diarrhea. Fluke eggs may be found only with a specific type of fecal examination. Your vet will prescribe specific treatment for flukes since they are not killed with traditional deworming medications.

Thelazia or eye worms are a problem in a few areas. They cause conjunctivitis and irritation of the cornea, which can lead to blindness if untreated. Your veterinarian removes the worms from the conjunctival sac with forceps.

Deworming Programs:
Sorting through the Choices
Deworming Products

Deworming medications can be classified into several large groups. Read the label to find the drug's generic name, and learn which drugs belong to the same groups rather than relying on brand names. In a rotation program, simply choosing different names or different brands of dewormers does not always mean that you are changing the class of dewormer.

Benzimidazoles are some of the most common dewormers in use today. Recognize them by their similar sounding names, most of which end in *-azole*. Examples include thiabendazole and oxfendazole. Febantel, a *probenzimidazole*, is metabolized to the benzimidazole form in the horse.

Benzimidazoles are safe and are effective against many different parasites, including large and small strongyles, roundworms, and pinworms. They are not effective against bots or the migrating larvae of large strongyles. Most do not affect the immature cyst forms of the small strongyles. The few exceptions to this include oxfendazole, which has some effectiveness against encysted small strongyles, and others at off-label doses.

The major disadvantage of using benzimidazoles is that small strongyles may become resistant to their effects. This resistance can carry over from one benzimidazole to another and may persist in a population of strongyles for many years, even after benzimidazole use stops. To overcome this problem, benzimidazoles are combined with other drugs, such as piperazine, or are used in a rotational program.

Not all small strongyles are resistant to all of the benzimidazoles. These products can still be an important part of your deworming program. The key is to check your horse with occasional lab work to be sure that the products you are using are doing their job.

Organophosphates, trichlorfon and dichlorvos, are most commonly used against bots. They are combined with other dewormers so that strongyles can be removed at the same time. Side effects that may occur with organophosphate use include diarrhea, colic, and irritation of the mouth, esophagus, and stomach. Problems are more likely when the drugs are given on an empty stomach. Be sure to feed your horse its regular breakfast when using this treatment.

Organophosphates are the main ingredient in products designed as feed-through fly control. These medicated feeds kill bots in the horse's stomach and then persist in manure, killing the fly larvae that breed there. Do not use medicated feeds at the same time that you give a paste dewormer.

Organophosphates should not be used in horses with heaves, as they may aggravate that allergic respiratory condition. They are also contraindicated for use late in pregnancy.

Tetrahydropyrimidines includes pyrantel, a dewormer that is very safe and is effective against many different parasites. In addition to its efficacy against ascarids, small and large strongyles, pyrantel is one of the few drugs that kills tapeworms. However, veterinarians must use this drug at a dose higher than that on the label to eradicate tapeworms.

Pyrantel is also available in a pellet form for continuous feeding. This product appears to control strongyles, ascarids, and pinworms effectively. A larvicidal dewormer such as ivermectin should be administered before beginning use of pyrantel pellets. Horses receiving continuous pyrantel therapy must still be given a separate treatment to eliminate bots.

Avermectins include ivermectin, a relative newcomer on the dewormer scene. Ivermectin is a safe and effective drug, but it is not a total replacement for the dewormers of the past. Many veterinarians fear that overuse of this product may lead to resistance by some parasites.

Ivermectin is one of the few treatments that kills the migrating stages of strongyles. Ivermectin works against adult small and large strongyles, pinworms, bots, and roundworms. These attributes make it an important part of your deworming program.

Piperazine is effective against adult small strongyles, pinworms, and roundworms. One problem with this product is the large volume required per dose, which may make tubing more practical for administration in adult horses. Piperazine is combined with a benzimidazole for tube deworming, since the piperazine kills the resistant small strongyles and the benzimidazole kills the large strongyles.

Several dewormers used in the past have been largely replaced by safer and better products. *Levamisole* has been used to treat lung worms, but is less effective and not as safe as ivermectin. *Phenothiazine* can have toxic side effects, and strongyles have become resistant to the drug.

Deworming Programs for Horses

Ask your veterinarian to help you design a specific deworming program for your horse. Housing, management, any clinical signs, and your horse's history are considered when a deworming program is designed. Your horse's age, its environment (pasture or stable, alone or in a group of horses), and its breeding status also influence the program.

You can deworm your horse with a paste administered directly into his mouth or with granules put into his feed. Dewormers can also be given through a stomach tube by your veterinarian. For the most part, the deworming chemicals in paste form are the same as those available as liquids to be given by stomach tube.

Administering a paste dewormer is not as simple as it may seem. First of all, you must accurately estimate your horse's weight to be sure you give the correct dose. You can use a weight tape to get a rough idea, but these tapes are not extremely accurate.

Your horse can use any food in his mouth to ball up the medication and spit it out. Therefore, medicate your horse just before you feed, when his mouth is empty. (Do not withhold feed, though). Thoroughly wash out the back of his mouth with a water-filled syringe before giving the medication. Slide the dispenser into your horse's mouth from the side, and deposit the medication far back on the tongue. (See chapter 5 for a complete description of opening your horse's mouth.)

Carefully read the label or question your veterinarian as to contraindications, side effects, and signs of toxicity for the product you've chosen. Deworming products should never be used in a sick or colicky horse, because they may worsen the condition. Check to be sure the product is labeled for use in your type and age of horse (pregnant mare, young foal) and that it works against the parasites you're concerned about. The label may not indicate whether the product kills immature larvae and migrating stages of those parasites, or whether those parasites could become resistant to the drug.

Discuss your program with your veterinarian even if you do all your deworming treatments yourself. Resistance patterns may have changed,

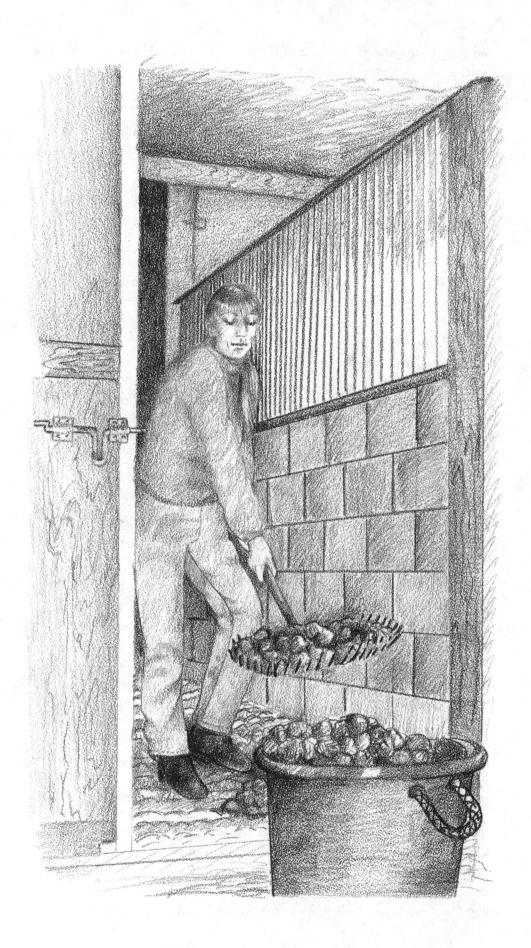

new drugs may be available, and there may be a problem specific to your area or to your type of horse.

Your main goal is to reduce the number of eggs passed, gradually reducing the number of parasites that infest your horse. Your deworming program should augment manure control, and not be used instead of good management. Without proper manure disposal, your horse will continually be reinfested with worms.

The young foal from birth to six months needs special attention. Strongyloides larvae can be passed from the mare's milk to the foal on its first day of life. Roundworms may cause problems in foals as young as six weeks. Both large and small strongyle eggs may be ingested, and their immature larvae begin to cause damage while the foal is still young and few eggs are being passed in its manure.

Deworm foals at monthly intervals. Start at six to eight weeks of age and continue to six to twelve months. During the second year you can go to bimonthly treatments.

Horses between six months to two years should be dewormed every other month. Roundworms and strongyles are of concern in these young horses. Most horses will begin to show worm eggs in their manure six to eight weeks after deworming. A bimonthly program will reduce the numbers of eggs and the potential parasite load of these horses.

Horses over two years should be dewormed every six to eight weeks; allow a shorter interval between non-ivermectin treatments than between ivermectin treatments. Your absolute minimum is quarterly treatments, but have your vet monitor fecal egg counts carefully if you choose to wait that long between treatments. The main concern for these horses are large and small strongyles.

Products that might be used alternately in this program are pyrantel, ivermectin, and a benzimidazole or piperazine-benzimidazole combination. If you don't use ivermectin, an organophosphate is necessary to take care of bots.

Pregnant mares should be dewormed every other month, both to keep the mare healthy and to reduce the numbers of eggs to which the newborn foal will be exposed. Several dewormers are safe for use in pregnant mares, including ivermectin, pyrantel, and many benzimidazoles. Carefully read the label to be sure the product is approved for this use.

Horses kept in groups must all be on the same deworming schedule. Group horses by age (weanlings, yearlings and two-year-olds, and older horses) in different areas. Isolate new horses until they have received a deworming treatment. Stall areas can build up large numbers of parasite eggs. A once-yearly stall scrub-down with Lysol or a similar product will keep eggs under control.

Controversial Ideas

Controversy, even among the experts, surrounds deworming programs. To rotate, or not to rotate? To tube deworm, or to use paste? New ideas are cropping up, such as seasonal deworming programs designed to kill the worms just before their peak egg-laying periods.

With effective products available in paste form, is there still a need for the traditional tube deworming? The answer to this question is that both tube and paste deworming are still a part of life for most horses.

Giving the same drug by paste or by stomach tube will have the same effect on the horse. However, you have probably experienced those times when half the container of paste ends up on the floor. It is also crucial to be sure that you have properly estimated the horse's weight. A tube deworming two to four times a year ensures that the drug is really getting to the place it needs to be.

What about rotational deworming? The argument isn't whether or not to rotate dewormers, but how often. The old school of thought says that a different class of dewormer should be used for *each treatment*. More recently, veterinarians have suggested that changing the class of dewormer *once every year or two* is a better idea. So far, neither argument has completely proven itself over the other, so follow your veterinarian's recommendation.

No matter which method of rotation you choose, remember that you are *rotating between classes of dewormers* (avermectins, pyrimidines, benzimidazoles), not between brands or names of dewormers (Cutter's, Telmin, etc.). Look beyond the brand name to find out what class of dewormer you are buying.

Monitoring Your Progress

Laboratory work will help your veterinarian to evaluate your deworming program. A *fecal egg count* is a microscopic exam of feces (manure) for parasite eggs. A yearly fecal done just before and again a few weeks after a deworming treatment will help to detect the presence of drug resistance. (You won't always see dead worms passed after you treat your horse because they partially decompose before they pass). Horses with mature, egg-laying adult parasites in their intestinal tract will be diagnosed easily this way.

Finding eggs in spite of regular dewormings makes us suspect drug resistance by the strongyles. A large number of eggs tells of poor management, both in deworming and in manure control.

Negative fecal egg counts don't tell the whole story. During the winter no eggs may be passed because small strongyles tend to be in their

dormant stage. And because of the long maturation time of large strongyles, horses may not yet carry the egg-laying adult stages in their intestine even though the larvae are inflicting their damage. If parasites are
suspected in spite of a negative fecal, further testing may be done (see
"Laboratory Tests" in chapter 9).

Easy Health Care
For Your Horse

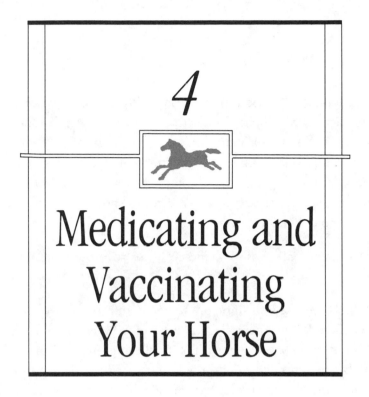

4

Medicating and Vaccinating Your Horse

Drugs and Medications for Your Horse

Like most horse owners, you have probably given your horse some type of medication this year. Perhaps he needed a little bute after he bumped his knee on a fence, or he may have had penicillin shots after a puncture wound.

The next time you casually reach for that bottle of penicillin, think twice: you may be better off with another choice—penicillin isn't always the first choice when your horse needs an antibiotic. Also, you might think of bute as just a painkiller, but it serves other useful functions as well.

Thousands of useful drugs are available for treatment of as many maladies. How do you and your veterinarian know which ones to use? Not only must the correct product be chosen, but also the proper dose, dosing interval, and route (oral or by injection).

Drug Types

When you look at a bottle of medication, skip the brand name and take note of the active ingredient. You can avoid needless confusion or dangerous mistakes by becoming more aware of the drugs you are using. There are no good or bad drugs. Every medication is helpful when it is properly and knowledgeably used. Some of the medications discussed here can be used only by your veterinarian. Yet you must know something about any medications your horse receives.

Biologicals include all those vaccines you use to protect your horse from disease.

Antimicrobials are used to fight off bacterial infections; they do nothing to stop viruses. While there are hundreds of different antibiotics, only a few are used on horses. Penicillins (including ampicillin, ticarcillin, water-soluble or aqueous penicillin, and long-acting or benzathine penicillin), tetracyclines, sulfonamides (trimethoprim–sulfa combinations), and the aminoglycosides (gentamicin, streptomycin) are some you may be familiar with.

Your veterinarian chooses the best antibiotic for your horse's problem by asking several questions. First, which organisms are commonly found in this type of infection? Second, what antibiotic is most likely to be effective against those organisms? Finally, the antibiotic chosen must go where it's needed. For example, the drug used to treat a joint infection must be absorbed well into the bone and joint.

In some cases, a culture and sensitivity test are done. A sample is taken from the infected area and submitted to the lab. The bacteria are grown out in the presence of various antibiotics. This procedure helps to find bacteria that have become resistant to a particular antibiotic, perhaps revealing why a stubborn infection hasn't cleared up in spite of regular medication.

Most antibiotics must be given by injection. An exception are the trimethoprim–sulfa combinations, which are available as tablets or paste. Be sure that you give your horse all of his medication as directed. You can cause an infection to recur or worsen by using an antibiotic at too low a dosage or for too short a time. Even if the problem appears to have cleared up, continue to use the medicine until it is gone or until you receive instructions from your veterinarian to stop the treatment.

Easy Health Care
For Your Horse

Anti-inflammatories stop pain in the process of their usual job of inhibiting inflammation. Inflammation is the heat, pain, and swelling that accompany the body's reaction to an insult. Inflammation is not the same as infection, although both can occur together. Infection results when bacteria or a virus invades the body.

The anti-inflammatory group includes corticosteroids and the nonsteroidal anti-inflammatory drugs, or NSAIDs. Most are available in both oral and injectable forms.

Side effects can occur with any drug. Many anti-inflammatory drugs, including aspirin, bute, and the corticosteroids, can predispose the horse to intestinal ulcers.

Corticosteroids are the most powerful anti-inflammatories available. Yet they're not used as much as NSAIDS, and for good reason: the accompanying side effects can endanger your horse's health. These drugs are such powerful inhibitors of inflammation that they may keep the body from naturally fighting off infection.

Corticosteroids are sometimes used to ease allergic symptoms. The drugs may be included in joint injections to relieve inflammation, but only after radiographs and other tests are done to be certain no fracture or infection is present.

Phenylbutazone, naproxen (Equiproxen), aspirin, dipyrone (Novin), and flunixin meglumine (Banamine) are well-known NSAIDs. Each works best in particular conditions.

Phenylbutazone is most often used for muscular and skeletal inflammation. When your veterinarian prescribes "bute" for your horse, it's not only for pain relief. Reducing the swelling may be just as important. For example, swelling contributes to the worsening of a bowed tendon. Ice and bute are used to reduce that swelling as well as to relieve pain.

Naproxen has fewer side effects than phenylbutazone. Its main use is in treating "tying up," a chronic form of muscle cramping and soreness.

Aspirin is used for long-term treatment of eye injuries in the horse and as an anticlotting drug in laminitis cases. Dipyrone is used for mild cases of colic. Severe colic symptoms will not respond to dipyrone.

Flunixin is often used in the treatment of colic. While the most obvious result is the relief of pain, flunixin also reduces intestinal spasms and attacks the toxins released during the colic episode. Flunixin is so effective that it can hide the symptoms of a severe colic. This could cause a fatal delay in treatment, if the horse appears better to an unknowing eye.

Dimethyl sulfoxide (DMSO) is an anti-inflammatory drug that can be used intravenously or topically. Veterinarians use DMSO intravenously to treat injuries to the brain or spinal cord. DMSO has the ability to penetrate the skin, carrying other chemicals along. For instance, mixing DMSO with an antibacterial ointment provides anti-inflammatory action and allows the antibacterial to penetrate.

Antihistamines, though not true anti-inflammatories, deserve mention here. Histamines are substances produced by the body during allergic reactions and other types of inflammation. Antihistamine medications might be used for horses breaking out in hives or for horses with heaves, an allergic respiratory condition.

Hormones are most often used to manipulate the reproductive cycle of the mare. Prostaglandins, progesterone, and others assist the breeder and veterinarian in enabling mares to become pregnant.

The anabolic steroids such as boldenone undecylenate (Equipoise) and stanozolol (Winstrol), are "protein sparing" hormones. Most are derivatives of testosterone, the male sex hormone. They are used to improve the attitude and appetite of sick horses, to improve body condition and muscle mass, and to stimulate weight gain. These products can cause infertility problems in horses used for breeding.

Analgesics (painkillers) include all the anti-inflammatories, as well as xylazine, detomidine, and the narcotics. Analgesics can be used before surgery or as a method of restraint. Only the NSAIDs are used for long-term relief of pain.

The narcotics include butorphanol (Torbugesic), morphine, and pentazocine (Talwin). Your vet might use a narcotic on your horse when severe cuts need to be sutured or when a standing surgical procedure is done.

Xylazine (Rompun, Gemini) is an analgesic and a sedative. It is used in situations ranging from easing pain in a colic patient to settling a fractious horse that needs his teeth floated. Detomidine belongs in the same family as xylazine. The effects of detomidine are longer lasting and more profound than xylazine's.

Local anesthetics provide analgesia in the particular area where they are injected or applied. Lidocaine and carbocaine are used before a wound is sutured to numb the area.

Sedatives and Tranquilizers include xylazine and acepromazine. Acepromazine is given by injection or in a powder form in the feed, and used for everything from calming a show horse for clipping to restraining a patient before general anesthesia.

Topical Medications

Topical medications include the huge variety of potions you can smear, spray, pour, or sprinkle onto your horse. They may contain anti-inflammatories, antibiotics, granulation tissue inhibitors, and antifungals, among others.

Topical medications will only do their job if the injury is thoroughly cleansed first. Each has a specific time and place where it is best used.

Easy Health Care
For Your Horse

Before you blithely smear any medication on your horse's wound, give your veterinarian a call to be sure that you are using the right product in the right place.

Ointments usually contain an antibiotic and are used under wraps or on open wounds that tend to become dry. Commonly used antibacterial ointments contain iodine (Betadyne or Providyne), chlorhexidine (Nolvasan), or nitrofurazone (Furacin). Ointments that contain aloe vera juice are useful for minor scrapes. Special ointments made for use only in the eye contain one or more antibiotics, plus or minus a corticosteroid.

Powders and Sprays that are antibacterial are useful for a variety of minor scrapes and cuts. Powders might be used on a cut that would tend to become weepy or dirty if an ointment were used. A spray could be easier to use on the sensitive horse that doesn't like its wound touched too much.

Liquid formulations are also available. Products labeled as a soap should be thoroughly rinsed off after use. Solutions do not have to be rinsed away but they might require dilution with water before use. The diluted solutions are ideal for flushing and cleansing wounds. Chlorhexidine, tamed iodine, and nitrofurazone are among the medications found in soap and solution form.

Strong iodine, or tincture of iodine, has an alcohol base and can burn the skin. Don't confuse it with the water-based, tamed iodine products. Strong iodine is used for disinfecting the foal's navel after birth, for some formulations applied to the sole of the horse's foot, or for blisters.

Scarlet oil is a special liquid used for deep cuts in the muscle. Its use is reserved for injuries above the hock and the knee only, since it stimulates tissue growth and can cause proud flesh (excess scar tissue) on the lower legs.

Sweats, Tighteners, and Poultices aid in the removal of fluid underneath the skin, in a joint capsule or tendon sheath. A sweat wrap placed over a puncture wound will help draw out infection and ease swelling (see "Bandages," chapter 8). Nitrofurazone ointment alone or with DMSO is commonly used as a sweat to reduce swelling.

Poultices are applied under a dry bandage or as a sweat. A poultice (also called a cataplasm or antiphlogistic) might be applied to the foot to draw out an abscess. A hot-water poultice can be made with magnesium sulfate (Epsom salts), mixed in the proportion of two cups per gallon of water, to draw out swelling.

Counterirritants include braces, liniments, paints, and blisters. All counterirritants will increase blood flow to the area they are applied. (See chapter 10 for more on heat as therapy.) Braces are used to rub down a

Medicating and
Vaccinating
Your Horse

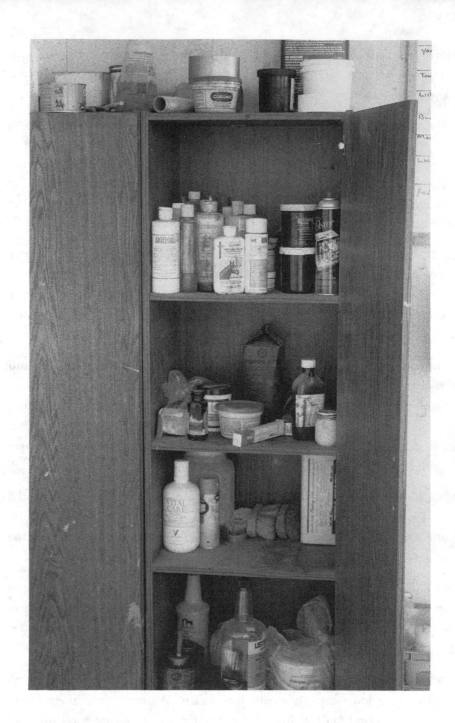

horse after a workout. Liniments will also increase blood circulation when they are massaged into a sore area. However, a bandage applied over a liniment creates a blistering effect.

Paints and blisters applied to the skin cause inflammation in chronic conditions. An increase in blood flow and heat is thought to turn the old, chronic condition into a fresh, acute one. Yet the "heat" that is created is not much more than skin-deep.

The strength of a blister determines how long it can remain on the leg. Severe burns can result from incorrectly using these products. Never

Easy Health Care
For Your Horse

apply a blister to broken skin or an open wound. Cross-tie your horse so that he can't rub the leg with his mouth (and so burn his lips and tongue). Do not use a blister on young horses, since their skin is easily irritated. Several cases of mercury poisoning in horses have occurred following the improper use of mercuric iodide blisters, so follow directions exactly.

Resting the horse is often recommended after use of a blister. Some veterinarians point out that it is the rest, rather than the blister, which makes the horse's condition improve.

Practical Use of Medications

Consider your medicine cabinet filled with various potions for use on your horse. Be sure you know when and how to use each product. Go through your cabinet, discarding any outdated materials or any with undecipherable labels. Discuss a first aid kit with your veterinarian, and decide which medications you will need to keep on hand. (See chapter 8.)

Always take the time to read a package's insert or the directions accompanying any medication. Do not change the dose or stop using a medication until you have specific instructions. If you don't understand the information, ask your veterinarian. Educate yourself about the side effects, indications, and contraindications for every drug you use on your horse. Some medications cannot be used in certain combinations, while others have dangerous side effects.

Be especially careful with medications you're using routinely and comfortably. Bute is one of the most useful drugs we have for horses, yet it can cause kidney problems or stomach ulcers when improperly used. Penicillin is also routinely given to thousands of horses, yet it can cause severe allergic reactions in some.

Drugs can be given by several routes, and certain drugs must be administered in specific ways. The choice may be limited by the type of drug, by how fast you need the drug to work, or by how long you want its action to last.

Oral: Drugs given orally (P.O.) must be absorbed by the digestive tract into the bloodstream. This route results in a longer delay before the drug begins to work, but is much easier for continuous treatment over several days. Some oral medications aren't absorbed into the bloodstream at all. These are given to treat infections of the intestine, since they stay where they are needed.

Injectable: Injections may be given by several routes. A subcutaneous (S.Q.) injection is given just under the skin. This route is commonly used in dogs and cats, but infrequently in horses.

Medicating and
Vaccinating
Your Horse

Intramuscular (I.M.) injections are given deep in a muscle. Several antibiotics, tranquilizers, and anti-inflammatories can be given by this route. I.M. injections take a half-hour or more to begin working, but their effects last longer than the same drug given intravenously.

If your horse requires penicillin injections over several days, you might end up giving them yourself. Wait until you are shown specifically how, when, and where to do so. Accidental injection of penicillin into a blood vessel can cause a severe, immediate reaction in your horse.

Intravenous (I.V.) injections act almost immediately. Accidentally injecting these substances outside the vein, or worse yet, into the adjacent artery, can have disastrous results. I.V. injections must be given by veterinarians or specially trained people only.

Topical medications are applied onto an affected area. Eye ointments, antibiotic creams, braces, and liniments do their work from the outside to the inside. Each has a specific place to be used, so don't try to use just one product for every situation.

Medications and Horse Shows:
Know the Rules

If you ever enter your horse in a competitive event, there's something you'll need to know: using the wrong medication, even unknowingly, can result in disqualification for you and your horse.

You'll need to find out what the governing body is for your particular competitive event and to get a copy of their rules. The American Horse Shows Association (AHSA) is one of the largest groups that publishes detailed accounts of unlawful medications. (See appendix for address.)

The American Quarter Horse Association (AQHA), the American Endurance Ride Conference (AERC), the North American Trail Ride Conference (NATRC), and each state's racing commission have their own, specific rules concerning medications. It's your responsibility to know these regulations and abide by them.

A large group of prohibited substances includes those that might alter the outcome of a competition: stimulants, depressants, tranquilizers, and local anesthetics. While many drugs, such as narcotics, are obviously forbidden, there are others you may overlook. These substances may simply be relatives of abused drugs, or they may mask the presence of an abused drug.

Masking agents are those that will cover up the presence of another drug in the horse's bloodstream. By themselves these medications are often harmless.

Some medications that you might watch include procaine penicillin, which causes a positive test for the anesthetic procaine; polyethylene gly-

Easy Health Care
For Your Horse

col, a masking agent that is present in many different injectable medications; and antihistamines, often outlawed because of their sedative effect.

What is acceptable? That depends on which governing body you ask. Some organizations have a "no drugs" rule, others allow only certain drugs at certain levels, and others have even broader rules. Likewise, penalties vary between organizations. As long as the issues remain controversial, you'll have to keep up with your organization's rule changes as best you can. Yet knowing that your ribbon was fairly won makes it all worthwhile.

Which Vaccinations Will Your Horse Need?

The variety of vaccines now available is mind-boggling. New diseases or new vaccines are constantly discussed. How can you decide what is best for your horse?

First, you need to learn the routine vaccinations used to prevent common equine diseases. Then you must determine whether your horse should be protected against any diseases peculiar to your area. Finally, you need to develop a common sense approach to evaluating new vaccines.

Consultation with your veterinarian is essential to keep up with information on new diseases and new products available. Even if you give vaccinations yourself, consult your veterinarian about a specific schedule for your horse. Every horse should have a vaccination program tailor-made for its age, use, and environment.

Vaccine Recommendations

Is your horse vaccinated against anthrax, botulism, or endotoxin? Which of the regional diseases is a problem in your area? How can you decide which, if any, of the new vaccines will be appropriate for your horse? Even if you get it straight today, there could be a new disease discovered or a new vaccine released next year.

You must develop a strategy for dealing with these unexpected occurrences. Using all the available vaccines is financially impossible and might have adverse effects on your horse. Omitting essential protection could bring even worse results, though.

Consider several factors while making your decision. What are the chances of your horse's being exposed to a given disease? Horses traveling to competitive events must receive more comprehensive protection than those staying in one place. Yet even the backyard horse must be protected against diseases that occur frequently in its area. If you hear of a new disease, don't start to worry until you've found out whether it occurs in your area.

Should you use new, improved versions of old vaccines? An improved version of an old vaccine may cost more, but could save you the even greater cost of treating a sick horse.

What about using a vaccine that can cause soreness, swelling, or even worse reactions? The risk of an inflammatory reaction must be balanced against the likelihood of your horse's contracting the disease in question. Reduce reactions such as pain, swelling, and stiffness after a vaccination by giving the injection in a hind leg rather than the neck. Exercise your horse for several days after the vaccine is given to keep the injection area from becoming stiff and swollen.

Should you use a new vaccine as soon as it becomes available? Unfortunately, some less-than-ideal products manage to slip through the cracks of testing and licensing. Ask your veterinarian to review the manufacturer's research data so you will know what to expect—regarding both the level of protection your horse will receive and the possible side effects that could occur.

To design a vaccination plan for your horse, first take note of the essentials: influenza, tetanus, and encephalomyelitis. Then make a list of the diseases that are a problem for animals of your horse's age and type. Add regionally important diseases to the list. Note how often boosters of each vaccination must be given. Finally, write down a specific vaccination schedule for the entire year. Follow your common sense and your vet's advice, and your horse will be well protected.

Use vaccination within a preventive health program. If horses must be grouped together, then keep each group separate from the next. Horses that are able to touch noses are more likely to spread disease quickly. Double fences or similar barricades between pastures and paddocks will prevent contact that could spread disease. Isolate new horses for two weeks before allowing them to join their herd mates.

Finally, avoid inadvertent transmission of disease on your hands, through shared tack and grooming equipment, or by neglect of general cleanliness.

How Vaccines Work

Your horse can receive protection against disease in several ways. They all involve injecting a modified form of a disease-causing substance into the horse.

When any vaccine is injected into the horse, specific disease-fighting proteins called antibodies begin to form. The horse is not protected immediately after receiving its vaccination because antibody production can take from three to fourteen days. A booster is a repeat of the same

Easy Health Care
For Your Horse

vaccination that is required to keep protective levels of antibodies circulating. Two boosters given three to four weeks apart are usually recommended the first time a horse is vaccinated. Foals may require more boosters since there may be interference from antibodies derived from the dam.

After his initial series of vaccinations, your horse's white blood cells retain a "memory" of how to make those disease-fighting antibodies for a variable length of time. Some products, like the influenza vaccine, stimulate only a short-term memory, and the horse requires boosters four or more times a year. Other vaccines stimulate much longer lasting immunity. If the horse is exposed to disease, its white blood cells are primed and ready to produce antibodies quickly, before the disease takes hold.

Your horse can be immunized with a toxoid, a bacterin, a killed virus, or a modified live virus vaccine. A *toxoid* is an inactivated toxin, (or poison) that is produced by bacteria. The tetanus and botulism vaccines are toxoids. A *bacterin* is made of inactivated bacteria. Some strangles vaccines are bacterins. *Subunit vaccines* contain just a part of a disease-causing organism. *Killed* (inactivated) vaccines use whole, killed organisms, while *modified live* (attenuated) vaccines contain harmless live organisms. *Recombinant* vaccines are made by taking a part of a disease organism and combining it with a harmless, live virus.

Basic Protection

Influenza

An outbreak of flu in a group of horses can bring disastrous results. The disease is very contagious, and every unvaccinated horse is at risk of becoming infected. Even with only a mild infection, a horse can be sick for two weeks. Although there are vaccines for influenza, the disease continues to occur frequently.

The equine influenza virus is not the same one that causes influenza in people, although both belong to the same family and cause similar symptoms. The equine flu virus attacks the upper respiratory tract (nose and throat) of horses.

Most severe outbreaks of the flu occur where large groups of horses are brought together at the racetrack, shows, or sales. After living in relative isolation at home, young horses are exposed to disease for the first time, and the virus quickly spreads. Horses can continue to shed the virus for a week after their apparent recovery, causing inadvertent exposure of other horses by unknowing owners.

In contrast to the human flu virus, the horse flu does not undergo frequent changes in its structure. Influenza A1 and A2 are the two basic varieties of the equine flu virus. The A1 variety is uncommon in North America, and causes milder symptoms than A2. All vaccines on the market today contain both strains. Several subtypes of A1 and A2 exist, and various combinations of them are present in different manufacturer's vaccines.

It is not necessarily good to have all subtypes present in one vaccine, since there may be a lower volume of each subtype and thus less protection. On the other hand, leaving out one or more subtypes may leave your horse susceptible to illness. Ask your veterinarian to recommend a specific product.

The flu virus spreads between horses by contact or coughing, and by your own accidental transmission—on your hands, for example, should you forget to wash, or on your shirt where a sick horse nuzzles you. Tack and grooming equipment also carry the virus between horses.

Symptoms of the flu begin one to five days after exposure to the virus. Fever and loss of appetite precede muscle soreness, a cough, and a runny nose.

The young horse affected with influenza can become very sick, and the virus may progress to the lungs. Older horses may have only the less severe symptoms of a cough and watery nasal discharge. Horses with a normal appetite don't need treatment other than rest. The symptoms last a week or two, then go away on their own. Sicker animals are treated with antibiotics and strict rest.

The live flu virus makes its way into the horse's body through the mouth and nose. Special antibodies are produced in the horse's nose as well as in its bloodstream. A vaccine injected into the muscle, though, causes formation of blood antibodies only. After three to six months, the horse's antibody level from a vaccination has dropped significantly.

Many horse owners mistakenly vaccinate for flu only once a year, leaving the horse unprotected for long periods. Show horses, racehorses, and any young horse that will be exposed to many other horses should receive two to four boosters each year. Be sure your horse receives a booster two weeks before traveling or competition.

A new type of modified live flu vaccine under development will be squirted directly into the horse's nostrils. It will stimulate antibodies in the nasal area that can stop the virus before it ever gains entry.

Strangles

Strangles is a disease that can mimic influenza in its early stages. Fever, loss of appetite, a runny nose, and a cough are its first signs. From there on, though, the diseases are quite different.

Streptococcus equi is the name of the bacterium that causes strangles. Strangles spreads between horses by contact, or on grooming equipment, tack, and human hands. As with the flu, a strangles outbreak is most likely to occur when groups of young horses are brought together.

The first signs of illness occur from three to six days after exposure. Fever, nasal discharge, and loss of appetite are just the beginning. The organism makes its way to the lymph nodes that drain the head and neck, and it multiplies there, forming large abscesses. At first you'll feel firm swellings under the jaw and at the throat latch; later these soften and rupture.

The horse's fever can run as high as 106°F, and the swelling in the throat area can be so severe that breathing becomes difficult (hence the name). Eating and drinking are painful, and the horse often holds its neck outstretched in discomfort. In uncomplicated cases, the abscesses rupture or are lanced, the pus drains out, and the horse proceeds on the road to recovery. Recovering horses may shed the organism for a month or more, possibly infecting other animals.

A few horses develop even worse problems. Infections of the guttural pouches can occur, which must then be flushed daily to remove the infection. (See "Inside the Ear," chapter 1, for a description of the guttural pouches.) The bacteria can also spread via the bloodstream to any lymph nodes in the body, causing internal abscesses that are difficult to treat and may be fatal. This serious complication is often called bastard strangles.

Treatment of strangles depends on the stage at which the case is diagnosed. Any horse with enlarged or abscessed lymph nodes is usually *not* put on antibiotics. This well-intentioned treatment will only cause the disease to be more prolonged and may result in bastard strangles. Although they look disgusting, the best course is usually to allow the abscesses to mature and drain. The high fever is treated with anti-inflammatories such as phenylbutazone. The enlarged lymph nodes can be hot-packed to draw out the abscess. An abscess that has softened might be lanced to allow drainage.

Exposed horses who are not yet sick have their temperatures taken daily and are watched for early signs of disease. Those that have a rise in temperature or other early signs of disease may be treated with penicillin. The dose used will be higher than that on the bottle, so be sure to follow your veterinarian's instructions exactly. Bastard strangles is a threat only if the antibiotic treatment is given at too low a dose or for too short a time.

Strangles vaccines have been available for some time, but are not used routinely. The first bacterins caused severe pain, swelling, and even abscesses at the injection area. At the same time, they didn't offer much protection against the disease. Newer bacterins have a reduced volume but still cause reactions in some horses. Some vaccine makers have turned to protein extracts of the organism, hoping to eliminate impurities that caused the reactions yet to retain enough of the disease-causing agent to stimulate the horse's immune system.

Like the flu virus, strangles bacteria enter the horse's body through the mouth and nose. The infection has already entered the horse's body and begun to cause its destruction before the blood-borne antibodies stimulated by vaccination come into play. A new vaccine under development will be administered through the nose and will cause the horse to manufacture antibodies there, stopping the infection before it progresses any further.

Which product you should use and how often you should vaccinate depends on your horse, where you live (whether strangles is common in your area), and the amount of exposure to other animals that occurs. None of the available vaccines claims to offer 100-percent protection against infection, but they do reduce the number of animals affected. The strangles vaccine might require twice yearly boosters for good protection.

Rhinopneumonitis

Rhinopneumonitis virus (rhino) can cause respiratory disease, abortion, or neurologic symptoms. Rhinopneumonitis is caused by an equine herpes virus, EHV-1. (The equine herpes virus labeled EHV-2 does not cause disease, and EHV-3 causes a venereal disease).

One thing that all herpes viruses have in common is their ability to live within the host indefinitely. Once a horse is infected with rhinopneumonitis, it seems that infection can be reactivated later when the horse is stressed.

Young horses are most often affected when they are brought together in groups. Rhinopneumonitis is spread between coughing horses or on the hands of unknowing people. An upper respiratory infection is a common result of virus invasion. Uncomplicated cases will resolve on their own in a week or two. Occasionally the illness will leave the horse susceptible to bacterial pneumonia or a guttural-pouch infection.

Another common result of rhino infection is abortion in pregnant mares. Some mares will carry their fetus to term, only to deliver a weak, sickly foal with slim chances of survival.

The neurologic form of rhinopneumonitis is less common. A high fever precedes the development of signs ranging from incoordination and weakness to paralysis. These horses may recover with nursing care, but it can take anywhere from a few days to several months.

Two different subtypes of the EHV-1 virus exist in nature. Subtype one usually causes abortion or nervous-system disease, while subtype two (sometimes called EHV-4) is most often the cause of respiratory infections.

There are two kinds of vaccine available now to help protect your horse from rhinopneumonitis. One is a modified live-virus vaccine, while the other contains a killed product. Whether killed or live, many rhino vaccines contain only subtype one, the major cause of abortions.

Easy Health Care
For Your Horse

Controversy rages within the veterinary community about whether some vaccines protect against disease at all, which forms of disease are prevented, how much actual protection occurs, and how long that protection lasts. Both the live and the killed vaccines are labeled for use to protect horses against respiratory disease. Only the killed product claims to protect against abortion. And none of the vaccines may be effective in preventing the neurologic form of the disease.

Many vaccines that are currently available contain only EHV-1 subtype one, the major cause of abortion. It's hoped that the two strains of virus have enough in common that vaccination offers some protection against subtype two, the cause of respiratory disease. Vaccines have recently been produced that contain subtype 2, or EHV-4.

While respiratory infection is not prevented, its severity is reduced and the length of illness shortened when any vaccine is used. For the competitive show or race horse, any advantage is better than none. Rhino vaccinations are not necessary for the adult pleasure horse. Watch for new developments, since research continues in the search for a better vaccine.

Tetanus

While all animals are susceptible to tetanus, the horse is the most sensitive species. Most horses are vaccinated against tetanus, but a few are still affected every year.

Clostridium tetani is the bacterium that causes tetanus. This organism is normally present in the intestinal tract. All that the bacteria need to begin an infection is a small wound such as a hoof puncture. *C. tetani* cannot cause disease unless it is protected from the air and is surrounded by dead tissue.

Even the smallest puncture wound is cause for concern in your horse, since it provides enough room for entry of the bacteria. Mares can contract tetanus after giving birth if a uterine infection occurs. Castration of the stallion occasionally leads to an infection, too.

Signs of tetanus can be seen any time from a few days to weeks after the wound occurs. Sometimes the horse's owner cannot recall that an injury has occurred, making the diagnosis of tetanus more difficult.

Tetanus-causing bacteria release a toxin that acts on the horse's nervous system, causing uncontrollable muscle spasms and paralysis. When the head is affected, the horse cannot eat, drink, or swallow, (thus the term "lockjaw") and may drool excessively. The animal may stand "like a sawhorse," its legs stiff and unmoving. The third eyelid tends to prolapse repeatedly, resulting in a characteristic "flicker."

Treatment of tetanus can be long and difficult. The horse's owner and veterinarian must be dedicated, especially to take the time necessary for nursing care. The horse cannot eat or drink, so nutrients must be provided

Medicating and
Vaccinating
Your Horse

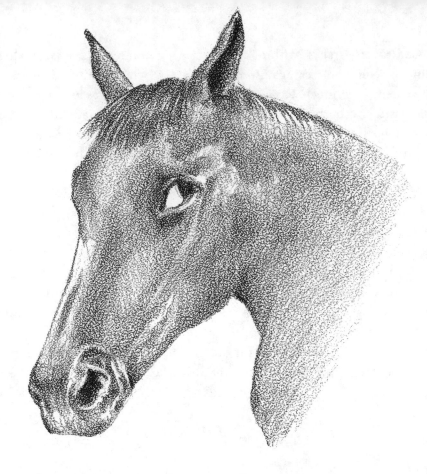

through a stomach tube or intravenous catheter. A padded stall is necessary since the uncoordinated horse may injure itself. Frequent turning of the down horse is required to prevent rub sores.

There are two types of protection against tetanus. Tetanus antitoxin gives temporary but immediate protection against disease for the horse that has not been vaccinated before. Antitoxin is sometimes given to newborn foals whose immune systems cannot yet produce antibodies against the disease. It is also given to adult horses that have no history of vaccination when they are at risk due to an injury.

Antitoxin is also given in actual cases of tetanus. Tetanus antitoxin will not reverse the disease's symptoms, since it cannot reach into the brain. The antitoxin is given to neutralize any toxin that has not yet reached the brain and to prevent symptoms from worsening.

Tetanus toxoid is the vaccine given to most horses to protect against the disease. Since the toxoid causes the horse to produce its own antibodies, the protection lasts longer than that provided by the antitoxin, but is not as immediate.

After the initial series of two vaccinations, repeat the vaccination

Easy Health Care
For Your Horse

yearly, as well as after an injury. Mares receive a booster one month before foaling, and foals are vaccinated at two, three, and six months of age.

Encephalomyelitis

Encephalomyelitis is often called "sleeping sickness" because of the effects it has on horses. This group of viruses attacks the nervous system, often leaving the horse dopey and depressed. There are several viruses found throughout the world that cause encephalomyelitis. Three of these are of concern in our country, and vaccines are available for them all.

Eastern, western, and Venezuelan equine encephalomyelitis (abbreviated EEE, WEE, and VEE) are three diseases that occur in North America. Each of the encephalomyelitis viruses has a unique life cycle, and each causes disease of a different severity.

As their names imply, the eastern variety occurs in eastern states, and the western one in western states. Venezuelan encephalomyelitis used to be confined to South America. The disease has gradually made its way up through Central America and Mexico to threaten the southern border of the U.S.

Eastern encephalomyelitis affects horses, people, rodents, and birds. Birds are the natural carrier of the virus, which is transmitted by mosquitoes to horses and people. Even though people can be infected with the EEE virus, you cannot get this disease from your horse. Horses and people are considered "dead-end hosts" of the virus. They do not carry enough virus in their bloodstream for a mosquito to pick up the disease there.

Because the symptoms in horses are often the same as those of rabies, the same quarantine precautions are taken until a definite diagnosis is made. Fever, depression, and loss of appetite are followed by confused behavior, teeth grinding, circling, and blindness. The horse usually dies within a few days. Treatment, if it is tried, is similar to that for tetanus.

Western encephalomyelitis is also carried by birds and transmitted via mosquitoes to people and horses. While the symptoms may be similar to those of EEE, horses affected with WEE often recover but can remain "dummies," with permanent brain damage.

Unless you live in a southern state or travel to other countries with your horse, you probably aren't going to be concerned with Venezuelan encephalomyelitis. The epizootic (epidemic-causing) form of the VEE virus causes severe epidemics in horses and people. The VEE virus can multiply in the horse's bloodstream and be present in large enough numbers that mosquitoes can pick up the disease directly from the horse. Thus, the virus can be transmitted quickly between horses and to people in the area. Even though VEE occurs rarely in this country, a severe epidemic could occur if the virus were to cross from Mexico or Central

America into the southern U.S. Routine vaccination of horses in southern states may help to prevent this possibility.

After his initial vaccination series, give your horse a yearly booster each spring before the mosquito season. In year-round mosquito areas, your horse might need twice-yearly vaccination. Foals in high risk areas are given more frequent boosters.

Regional Diseases and New Vaccines

Regional Diseases

Some diseases exist only in certain parts of the country, or are only a problem for particular groups of horses. While vaccines are available, they're used only on horses that require protection from those diseases. A few of the regional diseases, including equine viral arteritis, Potomac horse fever, and rabies, are discussed in detail in the following sections.

Botulism is another regional disease for which there is a vaccine. *Clostridium botulinum* bacteria cause this disease when their potent toxin is absorbed or released into the bloodstream. The result is paralysis and death. "Shaker foal syndrome" aptly describes botulism in foals.

Horses may acquire botulism by eating toxin-contaminated feed, by ingesting the bacteria that then release toxin, or through infected wounds. Foals may contract botulism through infected stomach ulcers.

Horses are affected by subtypes B, C, and D of *C. botulinum* bacteria. A vaccine containing type B, the most common form, is used in parts of the country with a high incidence of botulism and where the bacteria exists in high numbers in the soil. Since outbreaks of botulism in other parts of the country are relatively rare, vaccination is not recommended. Poisoning due to types C and D is less common, so vaccination is not done. Antitoxin against all three types of botulism is available, and although it is expensive, its use early in the course of disease yields a good prognosis for survival.

Anthrax is a deadly disease caused by the bacteria *Bacillus anthracis*. People, horses, and other livestock may be affected. Grazing horses ingest the organism, which enters the bloodstream and multiplies, releasing a powerful toxin that causes severe tissue damage, shock, and death. Anthrax occurs only in a few small areas of the country where the bacteria are found in the soil. The vaccine can cause severe inflammation after injection. It is only used where the disease is a problem.

Rabies

The sight of a horse with a neurologic disease is one you'll never forget. The horse may stand with its head tilted to one side, continually walking in circles; or it thrashes about, trying to get up without success. Milder cases may look slightly drunk, wobbling with each effort at walking, their legs not seeming to know exactly where to go.

Rabies is perhaps the most dreaded of neurologic diseases. Fortunately, it is less common in horses than in other animals. Horses account for only 1 to 2 percent of all domestic animal cases in the U.S. Yet horses in high-risk areas, where rabies is often diagnosed in wild animals, must be protected.

Rabies is transmitted by the bite of an infected animal. Animals most often diagnosed with rabies and most likely to bite your horse are skunks, raccoons, and foxes. Not all bites from an infected animal will cause rabies in the bite victim. Transmission of the virus requires that it be present in large numbers in the saliva, and that it be deposited on an open wound. The rabies virus travels through the victim's nerves, using them as a pathway to the brain.

The horse does not always exhibit signs of "madness" that we typically associate with the disease. Some horses become aggressive, attacking themselves or people. In others, signs of rabies can vary from colic to depression. The horse may become paralyzed or appear lame, disoriented, or sleepy. Eating or swallowing becomes difficult. Within a week, the horse is dead.

Diagnosis of rabies can be a challenge since the signs vary so widely. In areas where the disease is common, any horse with strange behavior should be suspected of having rabies. Taking precautions to prevent human exposure won't hurt even if a different diagnosis is made in the end.

Management of a horse suspected of having rabies depends on its location, its vaccination history, and whether known exposure to another rabid animal has occurred. Vaccinated horses that are bitten by a rabid animal are usually confined for observation. The unvaccinated horse that has been bitten must be destroyed immediately, or in some cases, quarantined for six months' observation.

What about the horse that shows signs of rabies, but with no proven exposure to a rabid animal? The same symptoms may be seen with rhinopneumonitis, encephalomyelitis, certain poisonings, and other diseases. Unless the cause of the symptoms is known for certain, the horse must be isolated from all other animals and people.

If you live in an area where wild animals are regularly diagnosed with the disease, then you should have your horse vaccinated. Rabies vaccine must be given by a veterinarian, and yearly boosters are recommended. Horse owners in areas where rabies is less common have something of a dilemma. Since the disease is invariably fatal, the cautious person will want to use the vaccine. Others may forego the vaccine to avoid the risk of side effects or because of the extra cost of vaccination.

Equine Viral Arteritis

Equine viral arteritis is so named because its symptoms are due to inflammation of the arteries. Many horses infected with EVA have mild symptoms that go unnoticed. In other horses, respiratory symptoms of red, puffy eyes and runny nose accompany a fever that lasts about a week. Sometimes a high fever, swelling of the legs and abdomen, and colic occur. Pregnant mares may abort.

The EVA virus spreads between horses by nasal contact. Stallion semen also harbors the virus. Some infected stallions become permanent carriers of EVA, showing no symptoms but infecting every unvaccinated mare they cover.

A blood sample can be taken for a screening test to check for antibodies to EVA. This test will be positive in vaccinated horses, in stallions that are permanent carriers, and in any horse that has ever had the disease. Have a blood test done on any stallion you intend to buy.

Vaccination of uninfected stallions will prevent them from becoming carriers of the virus. Any mare that is bred to a carrier stallion should first receive adequate vaccination. The EVA vaccine should not be used on pregnant mares.

If you own a brood mare or stallion, call your veterinarian for recommendations on the use of EVA vaccine. If you have any intentions of taking your horse to another country, have your veterinarian check that country's blood-testing regulations before proceeding with vaccination.

Potomac Horse Fever

The symptoms of Potomac horse fever begin so mildly that you aren't even aware of a change in your horse. A transient fever, sometimes accompanied by an unexplained buildup of fluid in your horse's legs, goes away in a day or two. But the tiny organism that causes the disease commonly known as Potomac horse fever (PHF) has just begun its destructive course.

A week or more after that initial temperature rise, your horse once again spikes a fever. Loss of appetite and severe depression soon follow. In some horses, recovery occurs without further symptoms. Others experience progression of the disease.

Ehrlichia risticii infects one of the horse's white blood cells called the monocyte. Mild enlargement of the lymph nodes occurs, then the organism travels to the intestinal tract, where *E. risticii* infects the cells lining the cecum and colon.

Some horses develop mild signs of colic, while others just look sick. Diarrhea is a symptom that actually develops in less than half of all cases. When it does occur, diarrhea can be severe and life-threatening. There is a massive loss of body fluids and endotoxic shock develops. The worst possible result of the disease, and another leading cause of death, is severe laminitis.

Once a horse recovers from PHF, it seems to be immune for a year or more. We now know that the disease is not confined to the Potomac River area, nor to river areas in general. Neither is "fever" an apt description of the illness. The traditional name, Potomac horse fever, is gradually being replaced by the more appropriate Equine Monocytic Ehrlichiosis or Equine Ehrlichial Colitis.

E. risticii, the organism that causes PHF, is a member of the rickettsia family. Since rickettsia can be transmitted by the bite of an insect such as the tick, the diseases they cause have a seasonal distribution and occur sporadically, in a hit-or-miss fashion, and do not seem to be directly contagious from one horse to another.

Diagnosis of PHF can be very difficult. It is uncertain whether PHF is actually spreading or whether it's just being diagnosed for the first time in many areas. While a blood test exists, a positive test only tells that the horse has been exposed at some time in its life. Two tests, taken two to four weeks apart, must be compared to show that the horse was recently infected.

E. risticii is very susceptible to the antibiotic tetracycline. This drug must be given intravenously, and its use is not without complications. Tetracycline has been known to cause severe diarrhea in horses.

Intravenous fluids are given to horses suffering from dehydration or shock. Other supportive and symptomatic treatments, such as anti-inflammatory medications, are given as needed. Until the final diagnosis is known most horses are isolated because of the chance that they may have a different, contagious disease.

Vaccinate your horse against PHF if you travel to shows or other events or if you live in an area where the disease has been diagnosed. After the initial series of two vaccinations, boosters are given twice yearly. If you live in an area where the disease has not been diagnosed and there is little in the way of horse movement, your veterinarian may not recommend vaccination.

New Vaccines

Expect to see several new vaccines on the market. Some of the vaccines mentioned here have recently become available; ask your veterinarian for more information.

Endotoxin protection may be provided by a toxoid–bacterin combination. Endotoxins are a part of the cell wall of certain bacteria that normally live in the horse's intestinal tract. Toxin is released when the bacteria die in large numbers or the intestinal wall is damaged. Many of the life-threatening effects of colic, laminitis, and other severe diseases are caused by release of endotoxins in the horse's body. This vaccine should help the horse to fight off some of the effects of endotoxin.

Lyme disease is a threat to people, pets, horses, and livestock in certain parts of the country. This tick-transmitted disease is caused by *Borrelia burgdorferi* bacteria. Horses affected with Lyme disease may suffer from intermittent lameness and fever. (See "Flies and Ticks," chapter 6.)

Equine infectious anemia is the disease that the Coggin's test can diagnose. The horse remains infected for life and has a cyclic reccurrence of illness, anemia, and weight loss. There is no effective treatment for EIA. Horses testing positive must be destroyed. The EIA virus belongs to the same family as the human AIDS virus. Because of their similarities, EIA is being studied in the hopes that new discoveries will help AIDS research.

Intranasal vaccines will one day provide protection against strangles, influenza, and rhinopneumonitis. Nasal sprays containing modified live organisms will have several advantages over injectable vaccines. Nasal vaccines will enter the horse's body in the same way that the actual disease gains hold. This method will allow the horse to produce local antibodies to fight off the disease before it gets into the bloodstream. Growth of the organism helps to stimulate greater antibody production, and it is hoped that protection will last longer.

Work continues to improve old vaccines, while several other equine diseases may someday be prevented with yet-to-be-developed vaccines. Diseases for which vaccines might someday be available include rhino virus, a cause of mild respiratory disease (not the same as rhinophneumonitis); rota virus, a cause of foal diarrhea; vesicular stomatitis, a virus causing severe blisters in the mouth; and contagious equine metritis, a venereal disease. There is even talk of a vaccine against strongyles.

Easy Health Care
For Your Horse

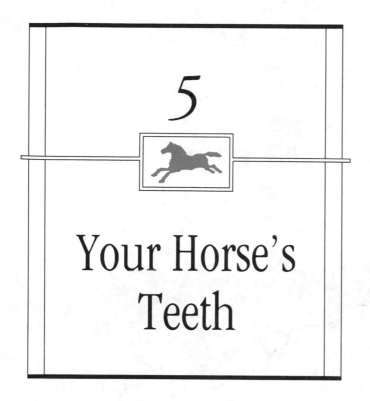

5

Your Horse's Teeth

Look in Your Horse's Mouth

Horse Teeth

Your horse needs regular dental care. Begin your understanding of the subject by becoming comfortable with opening your horse's mouth and learning about normal equine teeth.

The front teeth, or incisors, are used for grasping and tearing food. The upper and lower jaws each have six incisors. These are thought of as three sets, or pairs: the center or first; the second; and the outer or third set of incisors.

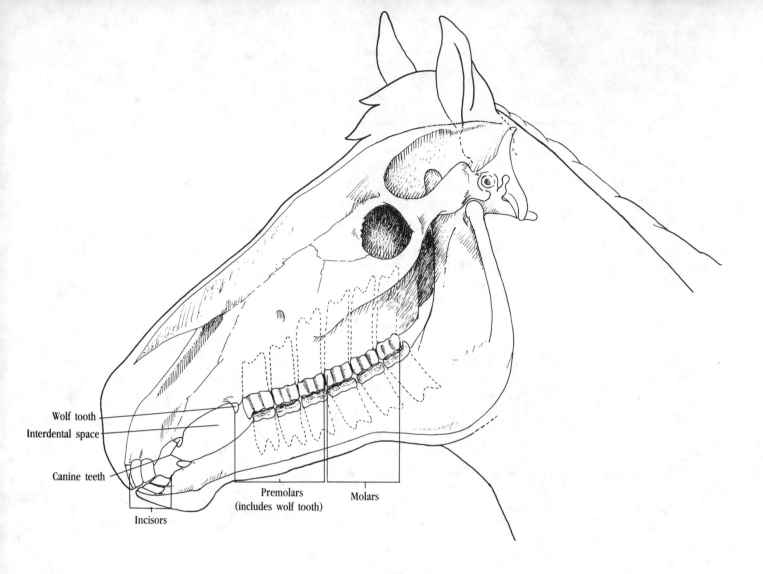

Wolf tooth
Interdental space
Canine teeth
Incisors
Premolars
(includes wolf tooth)
Molars

On each side, just behind the incisors, is the canine tooth. This pointed tooth is absent or very small in mares. Behind the canine teeth is a space several inches long (where the bit lies) called the interdental space.

Horses grind their food by using the three or four premolars and three molar teeth (the cheek teeth) on each side. The first premolar, or wolf tooth, is very small or nonexistent. Veterinarians routinely remove the wolf teeth before training is begun since this small tooth is thought to interfere with the bit. In some horses the wolf tooth falls out on its own.

How to Open Your Horse's Mouth

The interdental space provides you with a safe way to open your horse's mouth. First, be sure that your horse's halter is loose enough to allow his mouth to open. Stand at your horse's shoulder, facing his chest. Use one hand and arm to steady the horse's head. The other hand opens his mouth from the side.

Easy Health Care
For Your Horse

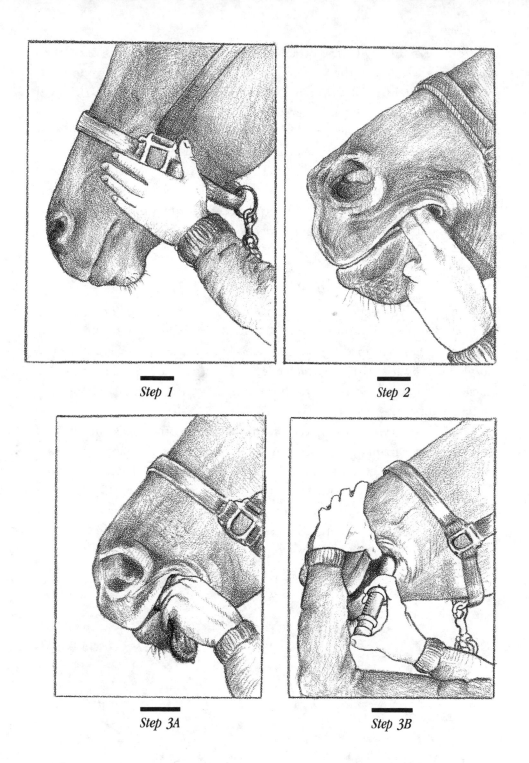

Step 1

Step 2

Step 3A

Step 3B

First, lightly place your fingers on your horse's lip, near the corner of his mouth. Gently wiggle your fingers until your horse stops fidgeting. Reach into his mouth through the interdental space and grasp his tongue. Pull the tongue out to the side through the interdental space. Now you can take a peek inside your horse's mouth. You will be able to see the surfaces of the incisors, which will help determine the horse's age. You can also see any problems with the front teeth. Look along the sides of the cheek teeth for sharp points. With one hand holding the tongue, you can feel for points with the other hand. Keeping your fingers parallel to the cheek, feel along the borders of the teeth for points. If your horse has a problem in the back of his mouth, though, your veterinarian will use a mouth gag to get a better look.

You will use the same procedure to administer paste dewormers or other medications to your horse, except that you don't need to pull out the tongue. First get your horse used to the feeling of your fingers in the interdental space, then slide in the tube of medication. Deposit the medicine far back on the tongue. If you don't feel safe working with your horse's mouth, ask your vet or trainer to help you learn.

Aging Your Horse by Its Teeth

A horse's teeth grow throughout his life. Although each tooth is fully formed, it lies within the jaw. Over the horse's lifetime, the teeth push outward. This has two important effects. First, we can tell the age of the horse by his teeth. Second, the horse needs lifetime dental care because of that continuous growth.

Baby teeth, or deciduous teeth, come in during the foal's first year of life. They are gradually replaced by adult teeth over the next five years. You can tell the age of a young horse by the number of deciduous and adult teeth that are present. A foal is born toothless or with the center two incisors just erupting. An easy way to remember when the baby teeth come in is with the phrase, "six days, six weeks, six months." The middle two incisors (top and bottom) have erupted by six days, the next two by six weeks, and the outer pair by six to nine months. The wolf tooth also comes in at around six months.

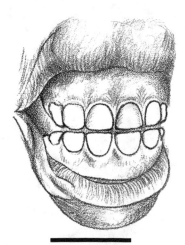

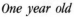

One year old

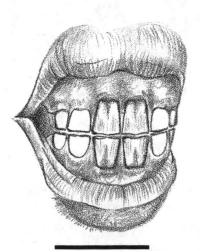

Three years old

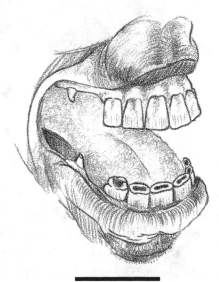

Five years old

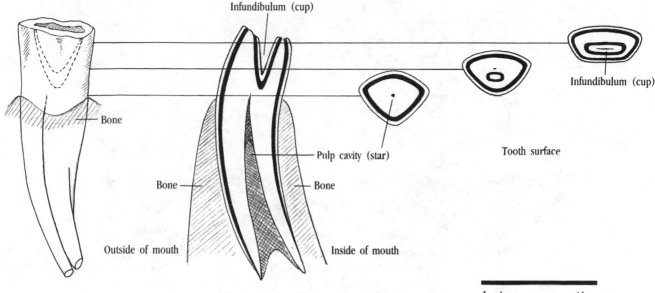

Infundibulum (cup)

Bone

Pulp cavity (star)

Bone

Bone

Infundibulum (cup)

Tooth surface

Outside of mouth

Inside of mouth

Incisor, cross section

Six months after each deciduous tooth has erupted, it has reached its full height. A yearling will have all three sets of deciduous incisors in place with the corner incisors at full height. Look closely to see the difference between adult and baby teeth. The deciduous teeth are smaller and rounded, with a narrow base. Adult teeth have a square top and are wide at the base.

Remember "two and a half, three and a half, four and a half" for the times when the adult incisors come in. When the horse is two and a half years old, the middle deciduous incisors will drop out and be replaced by adult teeth. The second pair will be replaced at three and a half years, and the outer pair at four and one half years. Six months after it erupts, each adult tooth has reached full height.

This means the center incisors which break through the gum at two and a half years will be at full height at three. A five-year-old horse will have all its adult incisors in, with the corner ones just reaching full height. The canine tooth has also erupted by five years. The young horse will have small bumps under its lower jaw that are the roots of the cheek teeth. This is normal and is no cause for concern.

Once all the adult incisors are in place, you must examine the wear on the tooth surface to gauge the horse's age. Once you know what to look for, this process becomes simple. Each tooth has a depression in it called the infundibulum, or cup. The infundibulum is not very deep, so as the tooth wears down, the cup disappears. The infundibulum is deeper in the upper incisors than in the lower ones.

At six years, the cups are gone from the lower middle two incisors. Remember "six, seven, eight" as the ages at which the cups disappear from the middle, second, and outer incisors of the lower jaw.

If all the cups are gone from the lower incisors, look at the upper

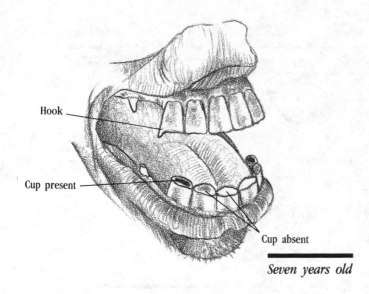

Hook

Cup present

Cup absent

Seven years old

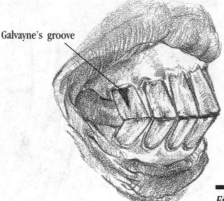

Galvayne's groove

Fifteen years old

teeth. Remember "nine, ten, eleven" as the ages at which the cup disappears from the upper middle, second, and outer incisors. Work at learning to age horses up to ten years before you try estimating older horse's ages.

To begin a logical look at a horse's mouth, first decide whether any baby teeth are present. If not, make a general judgment as to whether the horse is aged (with longer teeth that meet at a definite angle), or young (with square teeth that look almost upright). Next, look for cups in the lower and then in the upper incisors. Write down all your observation, then decide what the age might be. Practice on horses whose age is known.

For older horses the process becomes more complicated. Just in front of each cup on the tooth surface is a blackish line called the "star." This line does not look like a star at first, but as the horse ages it becomes more round. The appearance of the star on each incisor is used to estimate the horse's age from eight to thirteen years. The star appears on the lower middle teeth at eight, on the second lower incisors at nine, and the outer lower incisors at ten; it appears on the upper ones at nine, ten, and eleven years.

Changes in the Lower Incisors

Stage	1st incisor (middle)	2nd incisor	3rd incisor (outer)
Deciduous (baby)	6 days	6 weeks	6 months
Adult eruption	2½ years	3½ years	4½ years
Adult in wear	3 years	4 years	5 years
Loss of cup	6 years	7 years	8 years
Star appears	8 years	9 years	10 years

Easy Health Care
For Your Horse

Another aid in estimating age is the appearance of a "hook" on the upper, outer incisor. The hook appears at seven years, disappears at eight; it reappears at eleven years and disappears at fourteen. A line called *Galvayne's groove* appears at the top of the outer, upper incisor at ten years. The groove has moved all the way down the tooth by twenty years, and begins to disappear over the next ten years.

An old horse will have longer incisors that meet at a sharper angle than a young horse's. The chewing surface of the incisors becomes triangular in shape compared to the younger horse's oval surfaces. Once a horse is over ten years old, age estimates become very rough. Diet and chewing habits will influence the wear on the teeth. Some horses seem to have stronger teeth than others and will appear younger that they really are. A wood chewer or one that eats off the ground in a sandy area could have teeth that look very old.

Routine Dental Care

All horses need regular dental care. As the teeth wear, their edges become very sharp. Those sharp edges can cut your horse's cheeks and tongue. Badly worn teeth will keep your horse from chewing his food properly.

The horse's upper molars are not exactly even with the lower set. The upper arcade lies just to the outside of the lower. As the years pass and the teeth wear down, a pattern develops. The outer edges of the upper teeth and the inner edges of the lower teeth begin to develop sharp points.

Like people, horses don't always have perfectly aligned teeth or even wear patterns. Some teeth may wear faster than others, resulting in the appearance of a "wave" as you look down the chewing surface of the molars.

Left alone, sharp points and uneven wear will become worse over time. The horse's life span could be significantly reduced because of tooth problems. If the teeth receive regular care throughout the horse's life, these problems are minimized.

Dental Exams and Floating Teeth

Floating is the act of filing the horse's teeth. Special floats, or rasps, are made to be used on different sections of the horse's mouth. The points that are filed off do not contain nerve tissue, so the procedure does not hurt the horse. Still, many horses don't like the sensation.

Sharp points are not just a problem of the old horse. Young horses should have their teeth examined every six months. Sometimes a decidu-

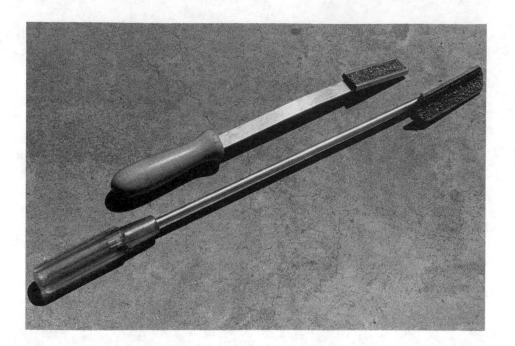

ous tooth is retained when an adult tooth erupts beneath. The "cap" must be pried off by your veterinarian. New teeth can be very sharp, so your vet might file off those edges just a little. If wolf teeth are present, the veterinarian removes them when the horse begins training or at about two years of age.

The horse from two to ten years needs a yearly dental exam. Most veterinarians look in the horse's mouth at the same time they conduct routine vaccinations or deworming. It's much easier to file off small points each year than to wait until they are a problem.

You can tell when your horse needs his teeth floated by watching him eat. Sharp points will cause him to chew very carefully or to drop his grain from his mouth, and he will gradually lose weight. (Next to parasites, sharp points are the main cause of weight loss in horses). Sometimes the horse will toss his head or chew at the bit more than usual when you ride.

Dental Care for the Older Horse

Like the young horse, older horses need a dental exam every six months. (The definition of "old" varies among horses, but as a general rule think of ten-year-olds as older horses). After ten years, many horses have developed a "wave mouth," sharp points, and other problems that need frequent attention. Once these patterns have developed, floating must be done more often.

By fifteen to twenty years, the horse may need a change in diet. Choose

Easy Health Care
For Your Horse

crimped or processed grain over whole grain. Be sure that hay is soft and green, without too many stems. If your horse has trouble eating hay, he may lose weight. In that case, feed cubes or pellets, which are easier to eat than hay; but continue to offer enough hay to keep the horse's chewing desires satisfied.

The horse with very bad teeth cannot eat pellets or grain. This horse needs a gruel or mash made every day. Pellets will make a nice mash without much effort. Just put the pellets in a bucket, fill it with warm water, and let soak for a few hours.

Problems of the Teeth and Mouth

Injuries and Infections

Several different injuries can cause your horse to drool excessively or to have trouble chewing. If the problem is not obvious, open his mouth and take a look. You might be able to find and remove the cause of your horse's problem.

Small chunks of wood, a piece of wire, or burrs (stickers) can become lodged between the teeth or under the tongue. Your horse will stand with its tongue hanging out or will constantly lick, chew, or drool. Open his mouth and look inside for the offending object. (Another common cause of drooling is choke; see chapter 9.)

A common injury to the mouth results from burrs or stickers in the hay. Some plants have extremely fine, needlelike stickers that can barely be seen. These penetrate the lips and tongue, causing ulcerated spots. Your veterinarian may need to shave the stickers off to get them out.

Tooth infection occurs when the root is exposed to bacteria. The roots of your horse's teeth lie within the upper and lower jaws. Several of the upper molars have their roots within the nasal sinuses. This means that an infected tooth could cause your horse to have a discharge from his nose.

Cracks or defects of the infundibulum are the cause of most tooth infections. Usually the problem is not noticed until it has become severe. The horse will have trouble chewing, and the problem does not resolve itself when the teeth are floated. In fact, the horse may resist having his teeth floated if an infected tooth is causing pain. Tooth extraction in the horse is not simple; it requires general anesthesia and a knowledgeable surgeon.

Fractures of the jaw are a common injury. The horse catches its upper or lower jaw on some protruding object and jerks its head away. You may notice that your horse is drooling, has an obviously deformed jaw, or just can't chew normally. Usually the jaw can be wired back in place under general anesthesia. A retainerlike piece of acrylic can help to hold the wires and protect them from harm.

A frustrating injury can occur if your horse jerks back on his halter when he is firmly tied. The halter lies over the facial nerve, which supplies movement to the lips. That sudden jerk can damage the nerve and leave your horse unable to eat or drink. Fortunately, nerve function can usually return if given enough time. The horse must be fed through a stomach tube in the meantime.

Paralysis of the tongue or throat is more serious. The causes can range from fractures of bones within the throat to botulism or other nervous system diseases.

Problems of Tooth Growth

Horses can be born with dental defects or they may acquire them throughout their lives. A horse can have a sore mouth and go off feed when the adult teeth are coming in. Retained caps must be found and removed to allow normal growth of the emerging adult teeth.

Some malformations acquired at birth cause the horse to have continual problems. Many abnormalities of the jaw can be inherited. The horse with "parrot mouth" has an overhanging upper jaw. You can see the condition by lifting the horse's lip. "Sow mouth" (monkey mouth, salmon mouth) is the opposite formation, with a protruding lower jaw. Parrot mouth and sow mouth can be inherited, so horses with these conditions should not be used for breeding.

Both these problems are not always limited to the visible front of the mouth. The entire jaw can be out of alignment; as the teeth wear, a large hook will develop at the back of the mouth where one tooth has no opposing member. The horse with parrot mouth or sow mouth requires frequent dental exams and floating throughout its life.

A common acquired dental problem is "wave mouth." The molars do not wear at the same rates, so you see a wave pattern as you look down the surface of the teeth. "Step mouth" is a severe form of wave mouth where there is a "step" in height between the molars. "Shear mouth" occurs when the upper jaw is a lot wider than the lower, making points on the outer edges of the upper cheek teeth. The lower teeth will have similar points on the inside edges.

Very old horses will have worn their teeth down to the gum line. The horse can do fine if a soft diet is provided.

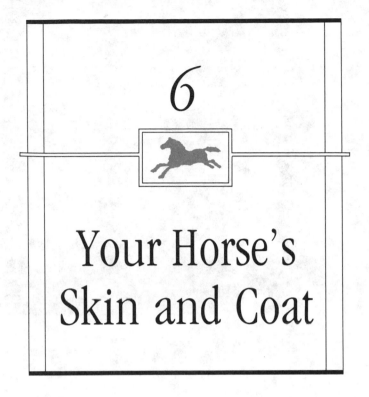

6

Your Horse's Skin and Coat

Grooming Basics

Grooming basics for your horse include bathing, brushing, picking the hooves, and cleaning the sheath of geldings. These are the essentials for good health. Chances are, you will add other tasks as needed for your activity—from pulling and braiding the mane to polishing the hooves.

Brushing and Bathing

Brush your horse lightly and pick his feet each day. Comb the mane and tail regularly and the job will be easy. Every horse must have its own

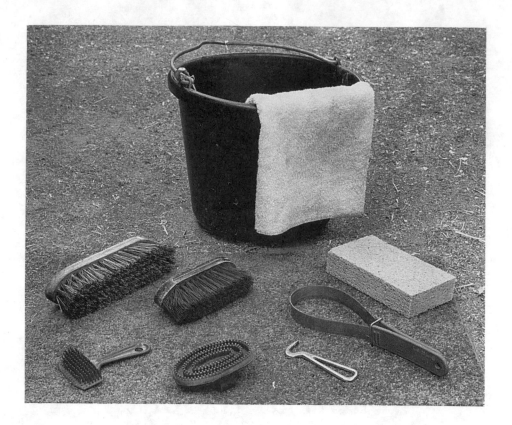

grooming equipment. Sharing brushes leads to transmission of disease. Among the grooming tools you'll need are a rubber curry comb, brushes (one stiff "dandy" brush and one soft "body" brush), mane-and-tail comb or hairbrush, sweat scraper, hoof pick, sponges, towels, and a bucket.

Before you ride, be sure to brush out any mud or dirt that would lie under the saddle, girth strap, or bridle. Dirt on the rest of your horse's body could also irritate the skin when the horse sweats, so groom him thoroughly.

There are entire books written on the subtleties of grooming (see appendix). As a general rule, though, start with your curry comb on the horse's body; next, use the stiff brush on the body, legs, head and ears (look inside for ticks in the summer); then finish up with your soft body brush. Use the mane-and-tail comb only if you don't have a show horse. Keeping a luxurious, long mane and tail requires separating out tangles with your fingers, since the comb will pull hair out.

Pay extra attention to your horse's lower legs during the muddy days of spring. Mud and moisture can cause a skin infection if it is not washed off regularly. The long hair growth of winter could hide a problem unless you brush the horse daily.

Although cold weather may prevent you from bathing your horse, you can still run a hose over the lower legs or wash them with warm water

Easy Health Care
For Your Horse

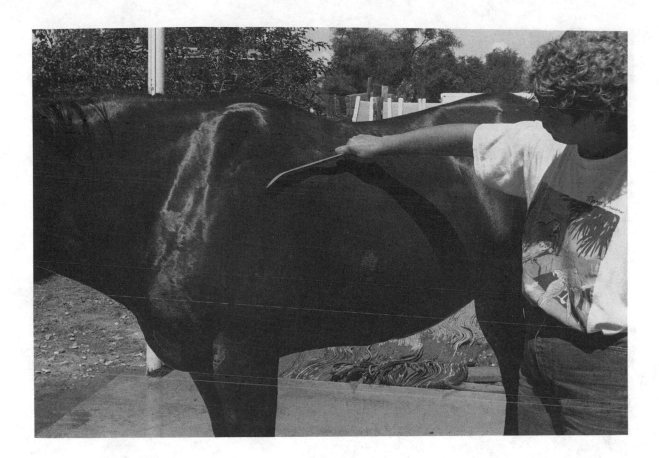

from a bucket. Allow mud on the horse's body to dry and then brush out the dirt.

Some horses need a bath more often than others. Use your common sense, and don't shampoo so often that you dry out the horse's skin. If your horse stays relatively clean with daily brushing, you don't need to bathe very often.

Proceed slowly if your horse is afraid of water or has not been bathed before. First, turn on the hose and let your horse see and hear the water running. Run water over your horse's feet, gradually raising the hose to rinse off his legs and then his body. Use a sponge to reach his head; most horses object to having a hose run over their face, and you might accidentally get water in your horse's ears.

Use a shampoo made for horses, or compare the ingredients lists on labels and purchase the equivalent human shampoo if it costs less. Mild, nondetergent soaps are necessary to prevent stripping away all the horse's natural oils. Rinse your horse until no trace of soap remains.

After a hot summer ride, sponge your horse's body or rinse your horse with a hose so the combination of sweat and dirt will not irritate the skin. First walk the horse until he's cooled out, then get him used to

Your Horse's
Skin and Coat

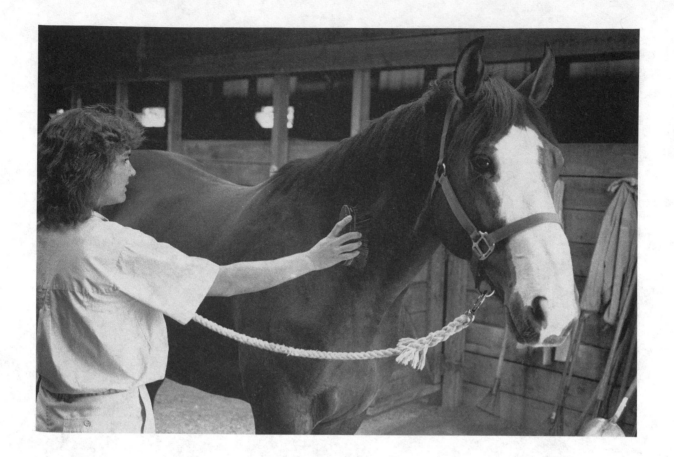

the water gradually. Start the hose on his feet, working your way up and over his back. In very hot weather, or after a strenuous workout, use lukewarm rather than cold water and avoid suddenly throwing cold water over the horse's back. Walk your horse until he's dry before you put him up.

Secrets of a Shiny Coat

You'll want your horse's coat to be shiny and healthy looking, but the glossy coat found on show horses doesn't happen overnight. The basis of a good coat is a balanced diet, frequent exercise, and routine health care that includes regular dewormings.

One important way to improve your horse's coat and skin is through vigorous daily brushing. Brushing removes dirt and excess hair. You can also help your horse shed out each spring with daily brushing.

If your horse stays outside in the winter, his thick hair coat will not look as shiny as the hair of a stabled, blanketed show horse. If you want a show coat in the winter, you must keep your horse warm with blanketing and a cozy stall.

Bathing your horse will remove dirt and add shine. Bluing is added to products for white or gray horses to add luster to the coat. Thoroughly rinse out the soap or the coat will look dull.

A conditioner can be applied after shampooing to replace lost skin oils. Polishes contain silicone, which increases the amount of light reflected from each hair. Polishes also make the mane and tail easier to brush out. Show horses have Vaseline applied to the muzzle and around the eyes for shine.

Several different feed supplements have been used to improve horse's coats. You can make your own or purchase a ready-made product. The main ingredients in most supplements made for skin improvement are fats or oils. Add a quarter cup of vegetable oil to your horse's daily feed to add gloss to his coat.

Cleaning the Sheath

If you own a gelding, you may need to clean his sheath regularly. The sheath is the area of skin that unfolds like an accordion when the penis is dropped to urinate. Waxy debris (smegma) builds up in the sheath and can irritate the skin. This irritation is one cause of a swollen sheath (other causes include insect bites and lack of exercise.)

The urethra is the tube within the horse's penis through which urine passes. Just inside the horse's urethral opening is a small pouch of invagination of the skin called the diverticulum. A small "bean" of smegma will form there and should be removed.

You can clean your horse's sheath yourself, or have it done by your veterinarian. Some horses are relaxed enough to drop their penis and allow cleaning without a fuss. Others require a tranquilizer to prevent them from kicking.

Once you are familiar with your horse's anatomy, you can clean the sheath without the horse's completely dropping his penis. Use your garden hose for a mild monthly flushing if your horse does not object. To clean more thoroughly, use a sudsy washcloth; reach up with your hand and be sure that you clean all the folds of skin. To get the bean out you must grasp the end of the penis and sweep the diverticulum with your finger.

Use plain water or a very mild soap, such as Ivory. Be sure that you rinse out every trace of soapy residue. Certain soaps can cause irritation and create a bigger problem than there existed before.

Some horses need cleaning only once or twice a year, while others create a greater volume of smegma and require cleaning more often.

Your Horse's
Skin and Coat

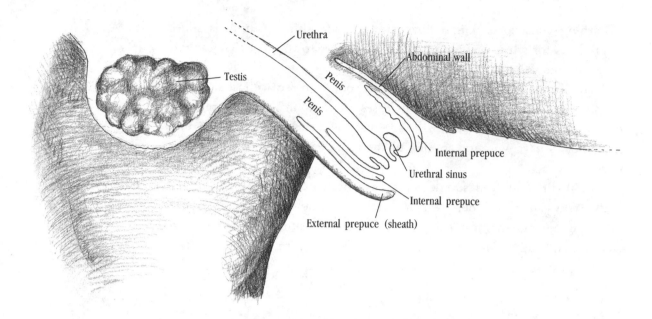

Urethra

Abdominal wall

Testis

Penis

Penis

Internal prepuce

Urethral sinus

Internal prepuce

External prepuce (sheath)

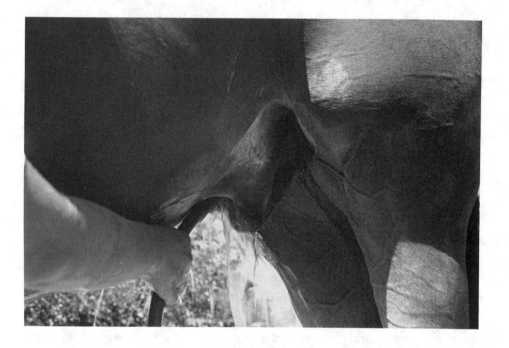

Geldings that do not completely drop the penis to urinate will need frequent cleaning. Use the amount of debris that you remove as a guide for when the next cleaning is needed. Have your veterinarian examine your horse if you find yourself cleaning the sheath more often than every month or two. Your horse could have an infection, or you could be creating a problem with too frequent cleaning.

Easy Health Care
For Your Horse

Causes of Tail Rubbing

We've all seen the rat's nest that results from horses rubbing their tails. Sometimes finding the cause of this annoying problem can be quite a challenge. Tail rubbing can have many causes, including parasites such as pinworms, mange, and lice; allergic reactions to *Onchocerca* larvae or *Culicoides* gnats; dry skin, or (most frustrating of all) the bad habit of a bored horse.

Check to see whether the tail is the only place that your horse is rubbing. If it is, you're more likely to be dealing with pinworms, dry skin, or a stable vice (boredom). The other causes of tail rubbing will result in hair loss in more than one place; check the legs, mane, and face.

Your veterinarian will diagnose the infectious causes of tail rubbing. If nothing turns up, you will have to contend with dry-skin problems or the bored horse. Use a mane-and-tail conditioner or a moisturizing shampoo made for horses (both available at your tack store) to ease the itchiness of dry skin. Turn out your horse if the problem appears to be boredom.

Skin Infections

My Horse's Hair is Falling Out!

Your horse has never looked worse, with patchy hair falling out all over his face, neck, and back. Only a few days ago, he had a little spot of hair loss over his eye. You thought he had just scraped himself. Now what can you do?

Hair loss can have many causes, including a variety of external parasites, bacteria, and fungi. Usually (but not always) itchy-skin problems are due to a parasite, while less itchy hair loss and scabs are the result of an infection. The most common skin infections are ringworm, "rain rot," and folliculitis. They can all look similar.

Fungal Infections: Ringworm

Everyone has heard of ringworm. Dogs, cats, horses, and people can all contract this skin disease. Still, it comes as a surprise to many people that ringworm is not a worm but a fungus.

Dermatophytes are fungi that infect the outer layers of skin and hair. There are many species. Each prefers a particular animal host, but most can live on a variety of animals (including humans) when the conditions are right. Warm and damp conditions encourage growth of the fungus, while heat and dryness inhibit its spread.

Ringworm can be spread either by direct contact or via brushes or blankets. It is usually spread from horse to horse, but may spread between horses and people. Young children are especially susceptible. Using good hygiene will keep you from contracting an infection and from transmitting the problem from one horse to another.

Young horses are most often affected with ringworm, since age brings a certain amount of immunity. In fact, a localized infection often will go away on its own if neglected for a few months. It is best not to wait to see whether this will happen, though. You'll risk its spread not only over a larger area, but to other animals and yourself as well.

The first thing you may notice in a horse with ringworm is hair loss around his eyes, face, and neck. Dermatophytes live in the outer, dead layers of skin and in hair follicles. Infected hairs become dry and brittle, breaking off close to the skin.

The infection can be mildly itchy, especially after the hairs fall out and leave a scaly patch. Ringworm in the saddle or bridle areas can become worse due to the constant irritation there.

Your veterinarian takes a skin scraping and loose hairs from the edge of an affected area. The fungus is sometimes seen by looking at the hairs under the microscope. The hairs can also be applied to a culture plate to test for growth of the fungus. The common belief that ringworm glows under a Wood's light (blacklight) applies only to certain types of ringworm. This test is not reliable in diagnosing the disease, especially in horses.

Localized, small patches of ringworm infection are easily treated with a shampoo, pour-on, or dab-on medication. Diluted, tamed iodine solutions or an iodine shampoo works well. Be sure to use a product recommended by your veterinarian. Continue treatments for a minimum of two to three weeks.

Treatment of ringworm works much better when you clip away the hair around the affected spots (always disinfect the clipper blades afterward). Horses with scabby crusts should be shampooed and have the scabs soaked off before the treatment is applied. Otherwise, the medication just sits on top of the scab rather than getting down to business.

Horses with widespread infections may need treatment with an oral prescription medication as well. Remember that even after the fungus is killed, the hair will still take time to grow back.

Don't forget to clean everything that touched your horse's skin, too. That includes brushes, blankets, halters, and saddles. When possible, wash or soak the items in diluted bleach (liquid chlorine bleach). Ask your veterinarian for a dust treatment (Captan) to use on items that can't be washed. Keep each horse's grooming equipment isolated or you will spread more than goodwill.

Easy Health Care
For Your Horse

Bacterial Infections:
Rain Rot and Folliculitis

"Rain rot" or "rain scald" are common names for a skin infection caused by *Dermatophilus* bacteria. (*Dermatophilus* is a bacterium, while *Dermatophytes* are the fungi that cause ringworm). If your horse is affected, his hair begins to fall out in big patches, especially along his back. It may be difficult for you to tell the difference between ringworm and rain rot. Your vet will take samples for microscopic examination and culture to determine the cause.

Rain rot occurs in horses that get wet and stay wet, so it is common in places like the Pacific Northwest. The combination of a wet, heavy coat, exposure to *Dermatophilus* bacteria, and some sort of skin scrape add up to a skin infection. Horses kept together may all get the disease since they share similar surroundings. Bacteria are spread by shared grooming equipment, tack, and flies.

Treatment begins by clipping hair over the infected areas, followed by cleansing with iodine solution or shampoo. All scabs must be soaked off so the medication reaches its target. Penicillin is used in addition to the iodine rinses for severe cases.

Disinfect all tack and grooming equipment as recommended for ringworm. If the problem recurs, you will have to find a way to keep your horse drier. A pastured horse may need access to a covered stall.

You can take measures to prevent rain rot in the horse that is predisposed to the problem. If your horse sweats a lot when you ride, rinse him with a hose following each workout. Frequent shampoos may help. Use a nonirritating shampoo recommended by your veterinarian.

Folliculitis is a bacterial infection of the skin. Pimplelike spots rupture, leaving crusty sore areas. Usually *Staphylococcus* bacteria are the culprit. Summertime sweating and irritation under the saddle and bridle set off the problem. Folliculitis can look like ringworm or rain rot, and like both of those, it can be treated with iodine shampoos. Sometimes antibiotics are necessary.

If your horse is prone to folliculitis, you will need to be meticulous in your grooming habits. Rinse him well after a sweaty workout, and get a medicated shampoo from your veterinarian. Keep your saddle pad and other tack squeaky clean.

Everything You Need
to Know About Scratches

"Scratches," or "grease heel," is a moist inflammation of the pastern area. Whatever the name, it is a messy problem. Oozing scabs and crusts along

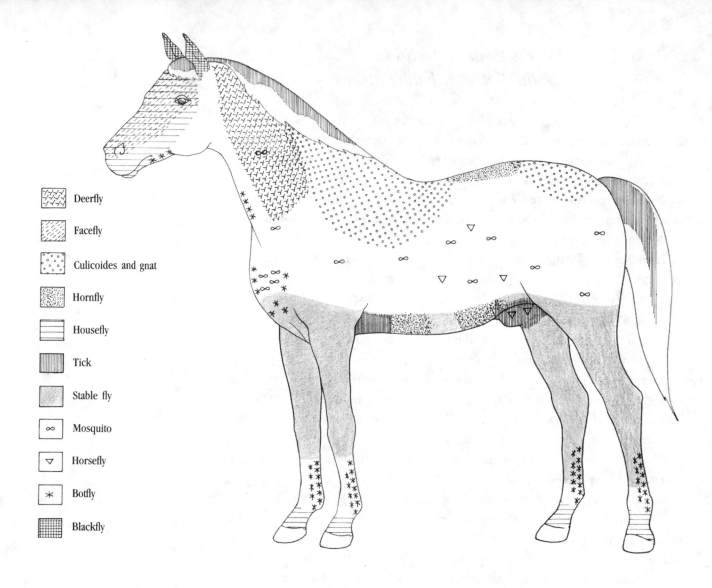

Deerfly	
Facefly	
Culicoides and gnat	
Hornfly	
Housefly	
Tick	
Stable fly	
∞ Mosquito	
▽ Horsefly	
∗ Botfly	
Blackfly	

with painful swelling of the pastern area can be caused by bacteria, fungi, or mites.

Staphylococcus and *Dermatophilus* bacteria, as well as the *Dermatophyte* fungus that causes ringworm, can all be involved in scratches. Mange mites can cause a similar-looking syndrome that is extremely itchy.

More than one organism can be present at the same time. Some veterinarians prefer to reserve the term *scratches* for only the staph infection; others lump all the causes together. No matter which organism is involved, the cause is similar. A wet, unclean environment combined with inadequate grooming creates a skin infection.

During the winter your horse's long hair may conceal an infection until it is severe. The first thing some people notice is lameness and swelling of the pastern. Closer inspection reveals the scabby infection.

Scratches can be difficult to get rid of, so be ready for aggressive treatment. At first, your horse's legs may be very sore. You must get all the hair clipped off so you can see and treat the problem.

Without daily cleansing, the infection continues under the scabs. Your goal is to gradually remove all the scabs. The easiest way to do so is with a long gentle scrub using warm water and iodine shampoo. Apply a poultice overnight to help soften the area.

Some veterinarians make up a cream mixture containing an antifungal, antibiotic, and anti-inflammatory, which ensures treatment of any of the infectious organisms that may be present and soothes the area as well.

Many horses are so sore and have such a buildup of exudate (serum, pus, and scabs) that it takes several days to get down to clean skin. Your persistence will pay off, though, so just stick with the program.

One of the most common mistakes is just swabbing on the medication without cleaning the area first. Remember that applying cream on top of scab on top of cream creates a big mess and doesn't solve the problem. Soak the leg clean before each treatment.

Treatment must be continued until you see pink, healthy skin with no scabs left. If you stop too soon, the problem returns. Keep reinfection from occurring by carefully grooming your horse every day, even if you don't ride.

A condition that looks similar to scratches but has a different cause is photosensitivity. Some plants (buckwheat and St. John's wort are two) can cause horses to have a hypersensitivity reaction to sunlight. Horses with photosensitivity are only affected on white areas of the legs and face. In contrast, ordinary sunburn usually does not affect the legs, while scratches does not affect the face and is not limited to white areas.

External Parasites

Itch, itch, itch . . . your horse has been rubbing against the stall door so much that his mane is all pulled out. It seems as if the condition happened overnight. The first thing to do is to find out what problem is affecting your horse. Hair loss or skin irritation are often due to an external parasite, skin fungus, or allergy. Allergic reactions to insect bites are common. Your veterinarian can help you determine what you're dealing with. The location and appearance help your vet narrow down the problem. A biopsy or skin scrapings for microscopic examination and culture might give a specific diagnosis.

A variety of parasites can get under your horse's skin, and all are manageable. The common parasites afflicting horses' skin include various flies, ticks, lice, gnats and mites.

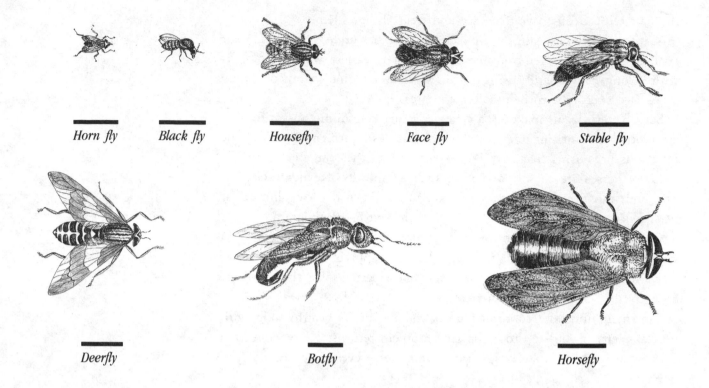

Horn fly   Black fly   Housefly   Face fly   Stable fly

Deerfly   Botfly   Horsefly

Flies and Ticks

Many different flies are nuisances to you and your horse. They range from small to large; some bite and others just bother. In addition to being a nuisance, many can transmit disease, so it's a good idea to keep all under control.

The housefly is the common little blackfly you see in your home. The biting stable fly looks similar. It lives in stables and paddocks, anywhere there is a pileup of manure. The stable fly gives a painful and bloody bite. House and stable flies transmit the *Habronema* larvae that cause summer sores.

The horn fly, a bloodsucker about half the size of a housefly, breeds in cow manure and attacks your horse when he's conveniently nearby. Horn fly bites cause scaly scabs on the horse's belly.

Face flies also breed in cow manure. They feed on the mucus draining from the horse's eyes, nose, and mouth. Not only are these flies extremely irritating, they also transmit the eye worm in eastern states.

You may have experienced the vicious, painful bite of horse and deer flies. These flies need water and mud for breeding and egg-laying, not manure like the other flies.

Blowflies lay eggs in wounds and on dead carcasses, which develop into the gruesome maggots you see later. Botflies lay their eggs on your horse's hair; immature bots travel through the horse's mouth to begin their winter life as stomach bots.

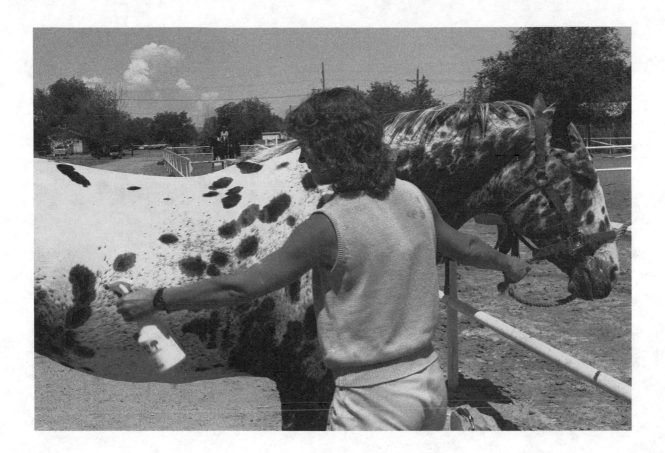

Blackflies are tiny biting flies. The female bites the inside of the horse's ear, leaving crusty areas. (You can help prevent the bites by wiping the ear with Vaseline).

Some flies breed in manure while others prefer decaying vegetation on animal flesh. Fly numbers can be kept down by daily removal of manure. Keep your manure pile as far as possible from the barn and riding area.

You'll probably make use of fly sprays or wipes that are made for horses. (Don't use anything on your horse that isn't specifically labeled for that use.) Apply fly spray to a cloth and wipe your horse's head and ears. Don't miss your horse's belly and sheath, too.

Occasional fogging or misting of the stable area may be necessary. Have professionals do the job for you or install an insecticide-dispensing system in the barn. Follow instructions exactly to avoid making you or your horse sick.

There are several alternatives to chemicals for fly control. For one thing, you'll rely less on chemicals if you keep manure picked up. Fly tape is an old, useful standby, and electric fly-zappers are noisy but effective. Jar, bag, or box fly traps containing a fly-attracting compound also work well.

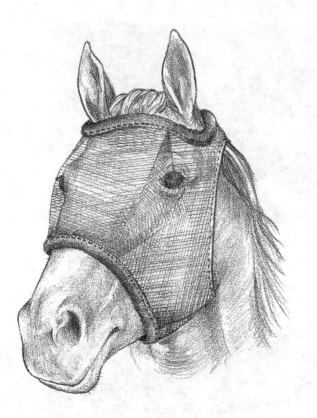
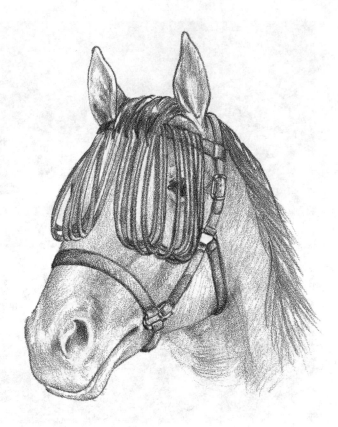

Consider biological control through the use of insects that eat flies. You can order these insects, which are tiny nonstinging wasps, from one of several suppliers (look in a summer issue of any horse magazine for their ads). Don't use fly sprays or baits on the premises at the same time or you will kill the wasps, too. Also, don't use feed-through fly-control products (see "Deworming Products," chapter 3), since the chemical residues in the manure will kill the wasps as well as the flies themselves. It's usually safe to apply fly spray to your horse while using biological control, since the wasps stay near manure where the flies breed. Follow your supplier's instructions.

Use a face net or a device that attaches to the halter to protect your horse against flies around his head. Most horses tolerate a fly mask without trouble.

Ticks, like flies, can transmit diseases and are irritating. A horse that has been shaking his head a lot lately may have a tick in his ear. Ticks latch onto the horse's body wherever a convenient spot is found. Lyme disease is transmitted by ticks in some parts of the country. Only certain types of ticks transmit Lyme disease, and not every tick is infected. You can minimize the chances of your horse's becoming ill by keeping ticks away and by removing those that do attach as soon as possible.

Regular grooming will help you find ticks and remove them from your horse. Unattached ticks range in size from a pinhead to a pencil eraser;

Easy Health Care
For Your Horse

after becoming engorged with blood, they enlarge into a rounder shape. Make a careful check after trail rides, and frequently look over all horses kept on pasture or in brushy areas. Many fly sprays are effective against ticks. Wipe the product into your horse's ears to prevent ticks from crawling in.

If you find a tick, you should pull it out. Do not use a match or kerosene to remove the tick; you don't need to kill the tick before you remove it. Gently grasp the tick's body next to the horse's skin with a pair of tweezers (not with your fingers) and pull straight out. Apply an antibacterial ointment to the area. If you are concerned that the tick head has broken off, simply observe the area for a few days for signs of infection. Infection resulting from pulling out ticks is rare, but if you are concerned, have your vet take a look at the area.

Lice and Mites

The thought of lice may make you shiver. Fortunately, horse lice don't infest people. Each species has a specific animal host and can't live anywhere else, which makes lice fairly easy to eliminate.

Lice are most commonly a problem in the winter and spring months, when the horse's coat is longest. The first sign of lice is itching and hair loss along your horse's mane, neck, and tail. If you part the hair and look carefully, you will see little whitish moving dots.

Lice are treated with a spray or powder insecticide, or with the dewormer ivermectin, a product that goes into the bloodstream so that the lice are poisoned when they bite the horse. Louse treatment must be repeated in a few weeks; the eggs present at the first treatment will have hatched by then.

All horses kept in the same area must be treated, regardless of whether or not they have symptoms. In addition, all brushes, blankets, halters, saddles, and anything else in contact with the horse's skin must be treated with louse dust (supplied by your veterinarian or obtained at the feed store). If you leave anything out, it will harbor the lice and eggs, and they will reinfest your horse. Since lice can only live long-term on the horse's body, you have a good chance of eliminating the pests if you are thorough.

Mange is caused by a little bug called a mange mite. You'll notice symptoms of severe itching, hair loss and scabs on your horse's face or legs. Some types of mange are transmissible to humans, but luckily for all concerned, mange is fairly uncommon in the horse. Mange requires two treatments, since, like lice, new pests will hatch from the eggs that survive the first treatment.

Mites are so tiny that they are invisible to the eye. Veterinarians diagnose mange by taking a skin scraping and looking for the mites

Your Horse's
Skin and Coat

under the microscope. In the unlikely event that your horse does contract mange, your veterinarian and family physician will advise you on how to prevent its spread.

Chiggers and straw-itch mites can also infest your horse. Both of these itchy diseases will usually disappear on their own if the source is removed. Chigger larvae ordinarily infest small rodents, and happen upon your horse when he travels through their territory. Adult chigger mites live in fields and woods. Straw-itch mites live in hay or straw and only incidentally infest you or your horse. Straw-itch mites will make their presence known soon after you've obtained a new load of hay or straw. Suspect this problem if you see bumps under your horse's hair at the same time that you develop an itchy rash. Horses don't seem to get as itchy as people do.

Gnats and Mosquitoes

Size is not proportional to ferocity among gnats and mosquitoes. The *Culicoides* gnats (also called midges, flies, or no-see-ums), are bloodsucking, irritating pests. They also transmit the skin parasite *Onchocerca* (see "Pests Under the Skin," below).

An allergy to the *Culicoides* bite, known as "sweet itch" or "summer itch," is a common cause of mane and tail rubbing. Occasionally horses will develop a reaction on the belly instead. Some horses that develop severe reactions to gnat bites must be locked away in a screened stall for comfort. Screens should be of extra fine mesh, since ordinary screen holes are bigger than the gnats.

Gnats come out at night, so bring the sensitive horse in before dusk and wait until the light of day to let him out again. Since gnats don't fly well in a stiff breeze, turning on barn ceiling fans from dusk until dawn will reduce their numbers. Using insecticidal sprays and shampoos and eliminating standing water where gnats breed also help control the problem. Spray your horse in the late afternoon for good protection all night.

The allergic horse's symptoms can be eased with antihistamine medication if necessary. A shampoo containing tar and sulfur could soothe the skin as well. Corticosteroids are used as a final resort.

Mosquitoes are the carriers of sleeping sickness (encephalomyelitis; see chapter 4), a fatal disease caused by a virus. The best way to keep mosquitoes away is to eliminate any standing water, but that is impossible in some areas. You can put goldfish into your stock tanks to eat up the mosquito larvae, and apply mosquito repellent to your horses daily.

Some equine parasites don't fit nicely into the traditional categories. We tend to think of internal parasites as those inhabiting the intestine (bloodworms and such), while external parasites include flies and lice. Yet there are two internal parasites whose symptoms are mainly related to the skin: *Onchocerca* and *Habronema*. Both these worms are transmitted by biting insects.

Hair loss, scabs, and itching along your horse's belly and forehead could be symptoms of an *Onchocerca* allergy. (Horn flies also cause lesions on the belly; often the problem is due to both parasites). *Onchocerca* are tiny worms that are transmitted by the *Culicoides* gnat. A gnat that bites your horse transfers the worms into his skin. *Onchocerca* larvae accumulate under the skin of the forehead and belly. Many horses have no symptoms of infestation, but others develop an allergic reaction to the parasites as they die.

Ivermectin is used for treatment of onchocerciasis. At first, the symptoms can worsen while the parasites die. Your veterinarian may administer an anti-inflammatory drug for a short time. The skin clears up a few weeks later, but your horse might need treatments several times a year.

Ulcerated tumorlike growths, called "summer sores," are the result of *Habronema* infection. Stable flies pick up *Habronema* larvae from horse manure. The immature stage of *Habronema* actually develops inside the stable fly.

The *Habronema* worm can infest the horse in several ways—it depends on where the stable fly deposits the *Habronema* larvae. *Habronema* deposited near the horse's mouth will descend into the stomach, where they develop into adult worms. Others are deposited on cuts, scrapes, and open wounds. Larvae invade the skin and cause an irritation reaction, resulting in a tumorlike growth. The horse's eyes, legs, and prepuce (sheath) are often affected.

Habronema larvae are killed by ivermectin. A growth that is very large must be surgically removed. You can prevent this problem by covering all wounds with ointment or a bandage.

What's That Bump?

The next time you find a lump or bump on your horse's body, take a closer look. Note the size, shape, color, and general appearance of the lump before you call the vet. Is the lump covered with hair, rubbed smooth, or bleeding? Is it firm or soft? How long has it been there, and is it growing in size?

A lump's appearance might tell the veterinarian what it is, but just as frequently a pathologist must examine a biopsy of the tissue for a diagnosis. Your daily grooming session is a good time to look at and feel your horse's skin. Fortunately, most bumps on horses aren't a big problem if you notice them early.

Nodular Skin Disease

Horses affected with nodular necrobiosis (nodular collagenolytic granuloma) are often affected each year at the same time. Nodules about a half an inch in diameter occur along the girth area, under the saddle, and on the horse's neck and back. The firm lumps are covered with normal hair, and you can feel normal tissues around and beneath them. The nodules are not itchy or painful unless they are under the saddle or girth, where constant rubbing creates a sore.

Nodular necrobiosis is sometimes called "protein bumps," but an allergy is a more likely cause. The lumps appear in the spring and summer. They tend to disappear in the winter or when the horse is treated with a corticosteroid.

Your veterinarian will take a skin biopsy to diagnose nodular skin disease. A local anesthetic is injected before surgical removal of the lump.

If the nodules are not bothering the horse, you can leave them alone. The nodules can be surgically removed if they're being rubbed raw by the saddle. If the horse has many nodules, corticosteroids are given during the spring and summer to help reduce their size and number. Unfortunately, this treatment doesn't always work.

Warbles

The lump created by a warble is about the same size as the those of nodular skin disease. In contrast, though, the warble lump occurs singly and has a small hole in its center.

A warble, or cattle grub, is a fly maggot. Cattle are the usual species attacked, but horses can also be affected. The warble fly (heel fly) lays its eggs on the animal, and the hatching larvae then penetrate the skin.

After several months of migration through the animal's body, the larva reaches the skin on the back, where it continues to grow, creating a small breathing hole through the skin. The warble emerges in the spring. The larvae falls to the ground and pupates into the adult fly.

Warbles should not be "popped" out of their hole, since an infection can result. Your veterinarian will surgically remove the warble from your horse. Fly sprays and other methods of fly control will prevent the problem from recurring.

Easy Health Care
For Your Horse

Warts and Sarcoid

Warts, which are common in young horses, have a characteristic appearance and location. They can occur singly or erupt in large numbers as gray, rough lumps that usually appear on the horse's lips and face. Although warts don't bother the young horse, they may concern the horse's owner. They generally go away on their own, no matter what we do. Warts are caused by a virus and can be transmitted from horse to horse by contact or by grooming equipment. Older horses are rarely affected.

Warts may become a problem for cosmetic reasons or because their size and number cause bleeding when the horse rubs on something. The warts can be frozen off. Another approach is to remove just a few of the lumps; this seems to cause the remainder to disappear more quickly.

A sarcoid can look similar to a wart, or it can grow and develop an ugly bleeding surface. Sarcoids can occur anywhere on the horse's body, but are commonly seen on the face, legs, and penis or sheath. Your veterinarian will recommend a biopsy with the tissue examined by a pathologist to diagnose the condition.

Sarcoids are thought to be caused by a virus. The sarcoid is a slow-growing tumor that is difficult to remove permanently. Although they aren't malignant in the sense that cancer can be, sarcoids do tend to recur after they're removed.

Sarcoids can be treated in several ways. One method of treatment is to remove the lump surgically, and then to freeze the surrounding tissue. Other cases are treated with a vaccine that is injected directly into the lump. This injection stimulates the horse's own immune system to attack the sarcoid. Two or more injections are given; after the second injection, the sarcoid may become more inflamed and look worse before it finally regresses. (See "Immune Modulators" in chapter 10.)

A warty sarcoid that is not growing can simply be left alone; surgical removal might tend to encourage the lump to recur, larger than before.

Cancer: Melanoma and Squamous Cell Carcinoma

Although cancer in horses is rare, two skin cancers do affect horses: the squamous cell carcinoma and the melanoma. Cancer is described as benign or malignant. A benign tumor is one that is not growing or spreading rapidly, while a malignant tumor can spread throughout the body.

A squamous cell carcinoma can occur on the face or penis and look very similar to a sarcoid. However, the carcinoma grows rapidly and becomes ulcerated. The result is a raised, rough-looking lump with a surface that bleeds easily. A tumor created by *Habronema* larvae (summer sore) can look like this, too. Your veterinarian will biopsy the growth to diagnose its cause. The squamous cell carcinoma can be effectively treated if it is removed completely and early in its course.

The melanoma is a tumor that occurs frequently in elderly gray horses. This tumor is usually a black lump seen around the anal area, under the tail, or less commonly, on the face. Most melanomas are benign, have a low incidence of spread, and grow very slowly. However, occasionally a melanoma can be extremely malignant, so the lump should be carefully observed and treated if there is any suggestion of enlargement.

Hives

Sometimes bumps require an emergency call to the veterinarian. Hives are an allergic reaction that occurs as suddenly appearing bumps. In severe cases, the horse's legs and face swell considerably, and itching can be intense. The horse's frantic attempts to scratch itself can result in further injury.

Mild cases of hives don't need treatment. In most cases, the reaction will usually subside on its own, but the horse can become very uncomfortable. Watch your horse carefully, and call your veterinarian if your horse seems uncomfortable or sick, if swelling covers the entire body, or if the face and neck are swelling considerably. Treatment of hives includes an injection of a corticosteroid, an antihistamine, and/or epinephrine, depending on the severity of the condition. Severe swelling of the throat area is potentially life threatening, but it is rare.

Hives can be caused by a number of allergy-causing substances, or allergens. A change of bedding or hay, certain drugs, fly sprays, and insect bites have all been implicated. Often the cause is never found.

A horse will occasionally have recurrent problems with hives. The best long-term treatment is to identify the cause and eliminate it from the horse's environment. If frequent use of fly sprays reduces the problem, then an insect allergy is likely. Sometimes symptoms occur with a change in feed or bedding. Try moving your horse from the barn to a paddock; if symptoms resolve, allergies to mold or dust are likely. If symptoms occur only during certain months of the year, then inhaled pollens might be the culprit.

Allergy testing can be done for horses just as it is for people. Allergy shots can be used to reduce the horse's reaction. Some horses need daily treatment with corticosteroids or antihistamines during certain seasons of the year.

Injury and Infection

Lumps can be caused by injury of infection. A hematoma is a blood or serum-filled lump that occurs after a foreceful blow such as a kick. Treat the small, fresh hematoma with ice packs and rest. The fluid will slowly be absorbed by the horse's body. Call your vet if your horse is lame, has a fever, or if the hematoma is larger than an orange. Large hematomas should be surgically drained by your veterinarian. Leaving the fluid there can lead to an abscess, or a permanent lump could result as the fluid clots and forms a scar.

An abscess is a pus-filled pocket of infection under the skin. A hematoma can turn into an abscess if the skin is broken, allowing infection to enter. Other abscesses are caused by a splinter of wood or similar injury that creates a small hole in the skin. Infection gradually builds up, but without drainage it cannot resolve.

A horse with an abscess is very sore and may run a fever. The lump will feel warm to the touch. If the abscess is near the skin surface, the lump will feel soft. Deeper abscesses will push out against the muscle and feel firm.

Treatment for an abscess starts with thorough drainage and flushing of the infected area. Your veterinarian will use a local anesthetic so the pocket can be explored for any remaining foreign material and all infection can be removed. You may be asked to continue flushing the area for a few days. Your horse will be given a tetanus booster and antibiotics.

Your Horse's
Skin and Coat

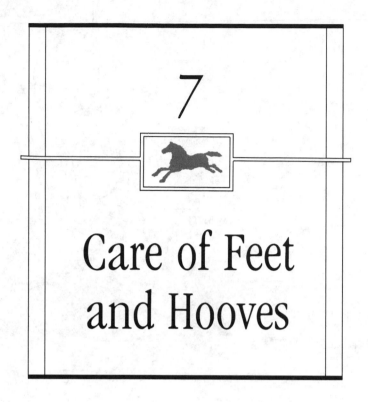

7

Care of Feet and Hooves

Daily Care of Your Horse's Feet

Your horse's feet could be the most important part of his body. A thousand pounds rests on these small foundations, with even more weight when the horse is moving.

As important as feet are to the horse, we don't pay much attention to them until something goes wrong. You should put as much work and thought into the care of your horse's feet as you do in to the rest of his health program. Your farrier (horseshoer) is as important as your veterinarian in keeping your horse healthy.

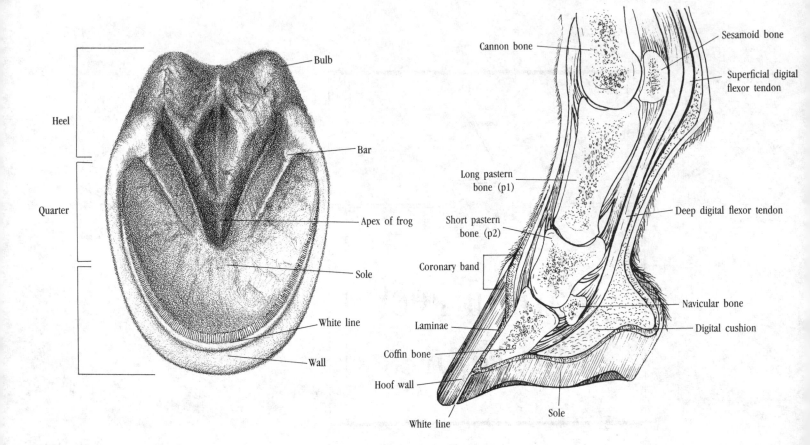

Heel

Quarter

Bulb

Bar

Apex of frog

Sole

White line

Wall

Cannon bone

Sesamoid bone

Superficial digital flexor tendon

Long pastern bone (p1)

Deep digital flexor tendon

Short pastern bone (p2)

Coronary band

Navicular bone

Digital cushion

Laminae

Coffin bone

Hoof wall

Sole

White line

Parts of the Foot

You'll need to know some basic anatomy so you can take care of your horse's feet properly. The hoof wall bears most of the weight and consists of dead tissue. The hoof wall grows downward from the coronary band (coronet) which lies between the hoof wall and skin. Parts of the hoof include the toe, the quarters, and the heels. The quarters are the thinnest part of the hoof wall. A thin, shiny covering called the periople extends down from the coronary band. This is the horse's natural protection against dryness.

Pick up your horse's foot and look at the sole, or bottom of the foot. In the center of the sole lies the frog; underneath the frog (inside the foot) is a spongy layer called the digital cushion. The white line can be seen at the junction of the sole and the wall. Horses that have foundered will have a widened white line.

Within the hoof lies the coffin bone, also called the distal phalanx or P3 by veterinarians. The coffin bone is suspended within the hoof by strong tissues called the laminae. Sensitive laminae contain blood vessels and nerves. The insensitive laminae are just under the hoof wall.

Examine your horse's feet to learn their normal shape and size. The angle of the hoof wall at the toe should equal that at the heel. The slope

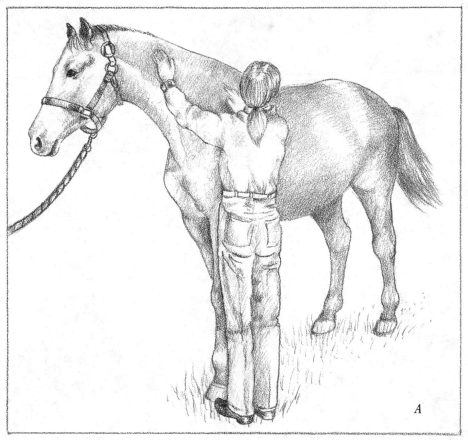

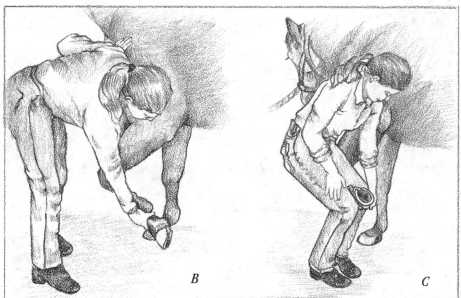

of the hoof wall should be about the same as that of the pastern. The normal hoof wall is smooth and even, and the length of the hoof wall is equal on both sides of the foot. The horse's right and left feet should be the same size and shape, but the hind feet are narrower and steeper than the front.

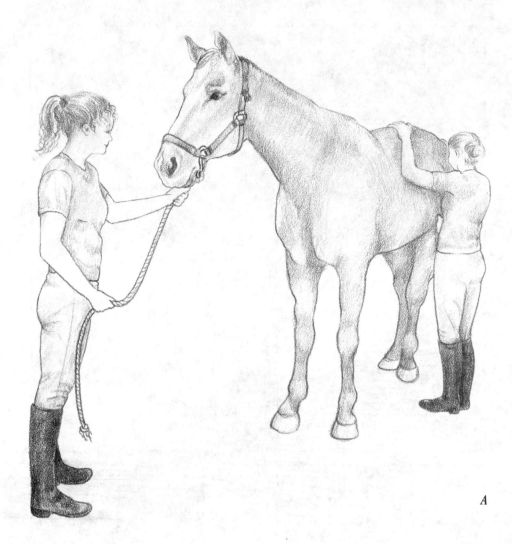

A

Trimming and Shoeing

Your daily grooming program should include thoroughly picking out your horse's feet. Look carefully next time, so you're aware of what is normal. You can then spot small problems before they become big ones.

Picking up your horse's feet can sometimes be embarrassingly difficult. There are several tricks that you can try to ease your effort. A little squeeze on your horse's chestnut (that leathery roundish thing on the inside of the leg) works like magic most of the time. Another trick is to gently lean on the horse's shoulder or hip to transfer his weight to the opposite leg. Pressing your thumb into the bulb of his heel or lightly pinching the flexor tendons might help, too.

Once you have lifted the foot, hold it so the horse is comfortable, keeping the leg under the animal's body. That way, you won't wrestle with a horse that is trying to balance itself.

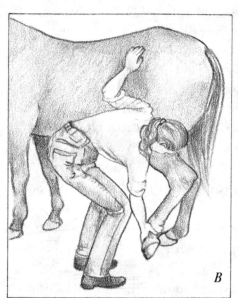

B

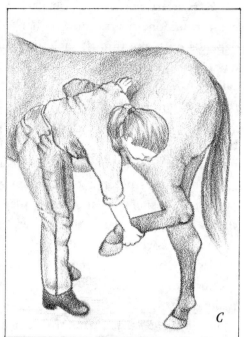

C

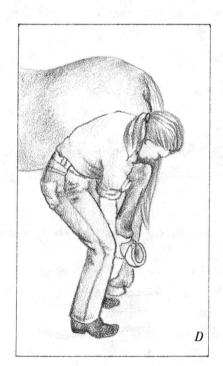

D

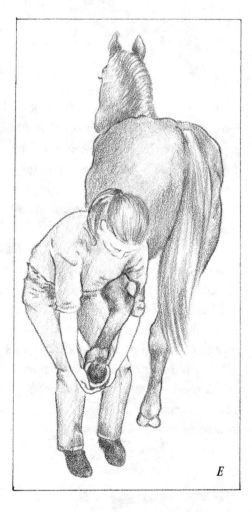

E

Care of Feet
and Hooves

How often should a horse's feet be trimmed? While the rule of thumb suggests every six weeks, each horse is a little different. The hoof may grow from one-quarter to one-half inch per month; its rate of growth depends on many things, including diet. Growth is slower in cold or dry environments. Set up a regular schedule with your farrier, rather than calling when you notice that the hoof is overgrowing the shoe. Follow a regular trimming schedule whether or not your horse wears shoes.

Ask your farrier to show you how to remove a shoe, and purchase the basic tools to do so. If you horse partially pulls off a shoe, you'll need to get it all the way off before one of the nails punctures the sole.

Do all horses need shoes? The answer lies in another question: why do horses need shoes at all, when they do just fine in the wild without them? The horse that is turned out on pasture can do quite well without shoes. Only when you begin to place more stress on the horse are shoes needed to protect the foot. A regular riding schedule, riding on hard ground, or the presence of certain hoof abnormalities or leg problems make shoes necessary.

During the winter months, when your riding schedule diminishes, your horse may be better off with his shoes pulled. The hoof can then expand naturally with each step, and the foot remains in healthy condition.

Choosing a Farrier

With so many farriers to choose from, how do you find someone you can trust to do the job? Start with word of mouth—call someone with a good reputation, who has done a good job with your friend's horses. Consider the farrier who cares for horses' feet at the stable where you ride. You need to be comfortable with the way the farrier interacts with your horse. The farrier should be comfortable with any questions you have about your horse's feet.

A farrier who has a good working relationship with your veterinarian is essential. While your horse may not have any foot problems now, you'll be glad to have that support if any problems should occur.

Should you choose a farrier who can do "hot" shoeing over a horseshoer who only does "cold" shoeing? Hot shoeing involves the use of heat to mold and manufacture special shoes, while cold shoers are limited to using premade shoes. If your horse requires a specially made shoe, then you'll need to find a farrier who is qualified to manufacture that shoe. Many horses do just fine with premade shoes on their feet, though. If you're not sure, follow your veterinarian's and farrier's recommendations on what is best for your horse.

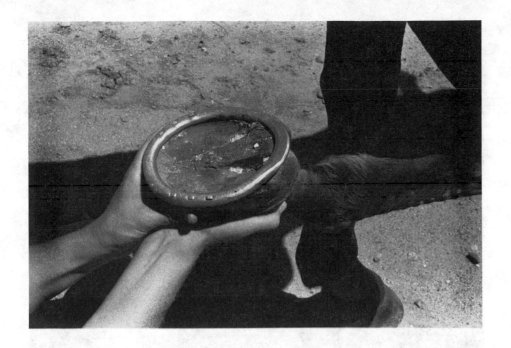

Should you choose a certified farrier over one who is not certified? Any farrier school will issue a certificate. In addition, the American Farrier's Association, which is open to any farrier, conducts an examination for AFA certification. Three levels of certification are possible—intern, certified, and journeyman. Certification at each level requires passing a written and practical test. The AFA maintains a list of farriers certified at each level (see appendix for address).

There are many talented farriers who are not certified by the AFA, however, so don't limit your search to that group. If your veterinarian and fellow riders have used a particular farrier for years and are happy with the work done, then you will probably be satisfied, too.

The Problem Foot

Dry Feet, Cracks, and Injuries

Minor foot problems include dry, flaky, or soft hooves, flat soles, and small hoof cracks. Any one of these can become a major problem, though, if they aren't tended to properly.

Dry, flaky hooves are a common problem. You can improve your horse's feet in two ways: from the inside and from the outside. The hoof wall is dead, like your fingernails, so you cannot put any moisture into it. You can prevent further moisture loss with hoof dressings, and help the hoof to grow out stronger with good nutrition. One cause of cracked hooves is too little trimming. As the hoof wall grows out it tends to flare and break itself off.

Care of Feet
and Hooves

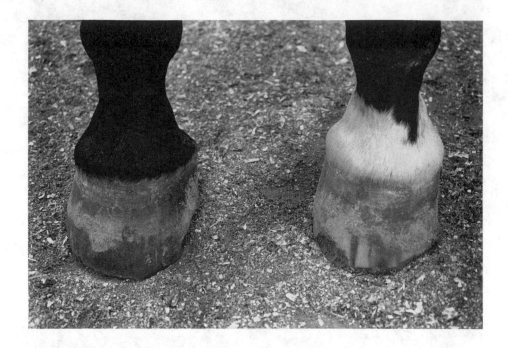

You can help hoof growth by making sure that your horse's diet is well balanced and of the best quality. Protein, calcium, biotin, and methionine are some of the nutrients needed for proper hoof growth. Try a supplement if your horse has poor-quality hooves in spite of a good diet. Supplements made to improve hoof growth usually contain methionine, biotin, and other vitamins.

Horses living in dry climates will tend to have dry hooves. If you live in a dry climate, allow your water trough to overflow a little. The horse will be forced to stand in the wet area part of the day, keeping his feet moist but not soaked. Constant mud or sandy soils will also dry your horse's feet. If the climate is wet, provide a raised area with good drainage somewhere in the paddock or pasture.

Hooves have a natural covering, the periople, which protects against moisture loss. Although some horseshoers want to rasp off this outer layer in the interest of good looks, don't let them do so.

Hoof dressings act by sealing in the moisture that is already present in the hoof wall. There are many different hoof dressings to choose from, and you may experiment with several before deciding on one that you like.

The main ingredient in any hoof dressing is a nondrying agent. Lanolin, fish oils, vegetable oils, and pine tar are commonly used. High-tech liquid polymers are available, which claim to last longer than the traditional treatments.

Preparations containing mild irritants are intended for use on the coronary band, in the theory that the irritation will stimulate faster growth.

Easy Health Care
For Your Horse

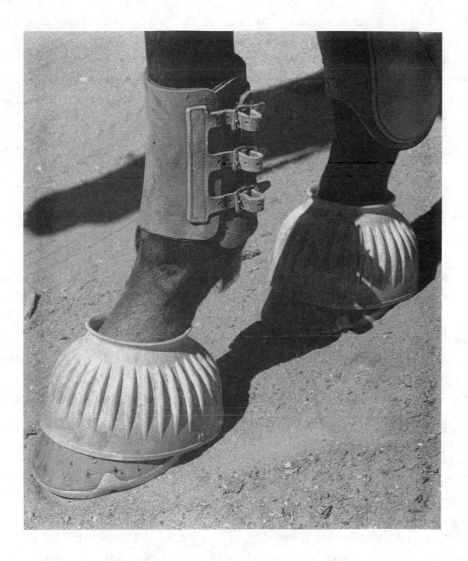

Pine tar, iodine, and turpentine are irritants found in hoof dressings. Unfortunately, most irritants are also drying agents, which have the opposite effect to what you want to use on the hoof wall.

Soles that are too soft and moist are as bothersome as dry hooves (see "Soft Soles, Sole Bruises, and Abscesses," below). Soft soles bruise easily and can be prone to infection.

Hoof wall injuries range from small cracks to cuts and abrasions of the coronary band. Prevent a small hoof crack from becoming a problem by having your farrier tend to it at once. A bar shoe or clips will help remove stress from the area so new hoof can grow out without perpetuating the crack.

Deep cracks will bleed or make your horse lame. Your farrier and veterinarian will work together to repair deep cracks. The crack can be sewn together, then held in place with an acrylic or fiberglass patch. A bar shoe will provide further strength.

Injuries to the coronary band can be serious. This band of tissue contains the cells that grow out to become the hoof wall. If the tissues are disturbed, subsequent hoof growth will be abnormal. To be safe, have your vet take a look at any injury in the coronary band area. Deep cuts will require intensive care. Sometimes a cast is applied to prevent movement and to allow the injury to heal in place.

Thrush and Canker

Thrush and canker are infections of the foot. Mild thrush is a common problem. You'll notice foul-smelling black material in the grooves of the frog when you pick out your horse's feet.

Thrush occurs in horses whose feet are constantly wet. Horses left in muddy paddocks or infrequently cleaned stalls are susceptible. If you notice thrush early in its course, treatment is easier.

Medication is used to kill the thrush-causing bacteria and to dry the sole and frog. Many different substances, including liquid chlorine bleach, strong iodine, and formaldehyde, will kill the bacteria. You must pick your horse's feet and apply the medication daily or the problem will recur. Since the medications are caustic, wear gloves and don't allow the liquid to drip on you or on your horse.

Canker is also an infection of the sole and frog, but it is much more serious than thrush. Canker results in lameness because it infects the deep tissues. You'll see a warty, whitish growth on the sole and frog. Treatment of canker should be left to your veterinarian, since improper removal of the material could make the infection much worse. The infected tissue will have to be surgically removed with the horse under a general anesthetic.

Lameness and the Foot

Most veterinarians will agree that foot problems are a common cause of lameness. Yet the scope of problems found in this small area is quite large. The balance of the horse's foot affects the way stress is placed on the entire leg. Many lameness problems can be traced to a previously existing abnormality of the foot.

Spotting Foot Abnormalities

Abnormal shape, growth, or balance of the foot can be a cause or a result of a lameness. Lameness due to a problem higher up on the leg may improve through a change in trimming or shoeing.

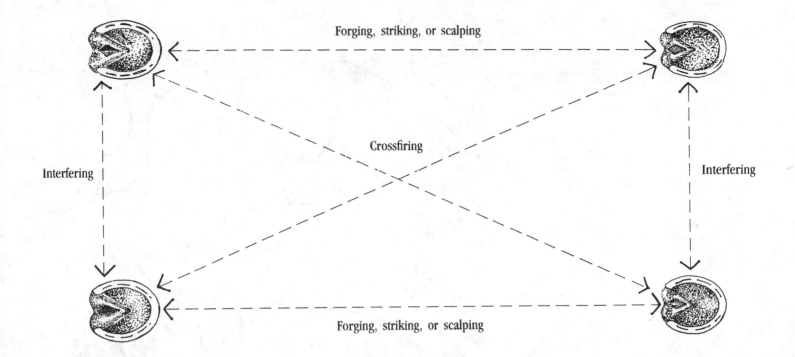

Forging, striking, or scalping

Crossfiring

Interfering

Interfering

Forging, striking, or scalping

Some horses develop problems due to poor conformation. Horses with a toe-out conformation may interfere, or hit themselves with opposing legs at each stride. Careful trimming and shoeing can help them regain a normal stride and prevent self-inflicted injury.

Other cases involve forging or overreaching, when the horse strikes its forefeet with the hind feet. Appropriate trimming and shoeing help minimize this problem.

Under-run heels occur when the angle at the toe is more than five degrees steeper than that at the heel. Their cause is often improper trimming.

Contracted heels occur when the frog width is less than two-thirds its length. Contracted heels result from improper hoof expansion. The hoof expands with each stride as the horse's weight bears down on the leg. When the foot or heel is painful, the horse does not bear full weight on the area and contraction results.

The horse with a long-term lameness will place less weight on the lame foot with each stride. Over time, that foot will become smaller than its opposite. Suspect a chronic lameness problem if you can easily spot a difference in size between a horse's left and right feet.

Sheared heels are defined as a difference in length of the hoof wall between the inside and outside of the foot. Sheared heels are associated with many different problems, including navicular disease.

A club foot is one that is club-shaped, or has an abnormally steep hoof wall. The cause of a club foot is usually a contracted (shortened) flexor tendon. Very young horses can sometimes be corrected, but the condition

Care of Feet
and Hooves

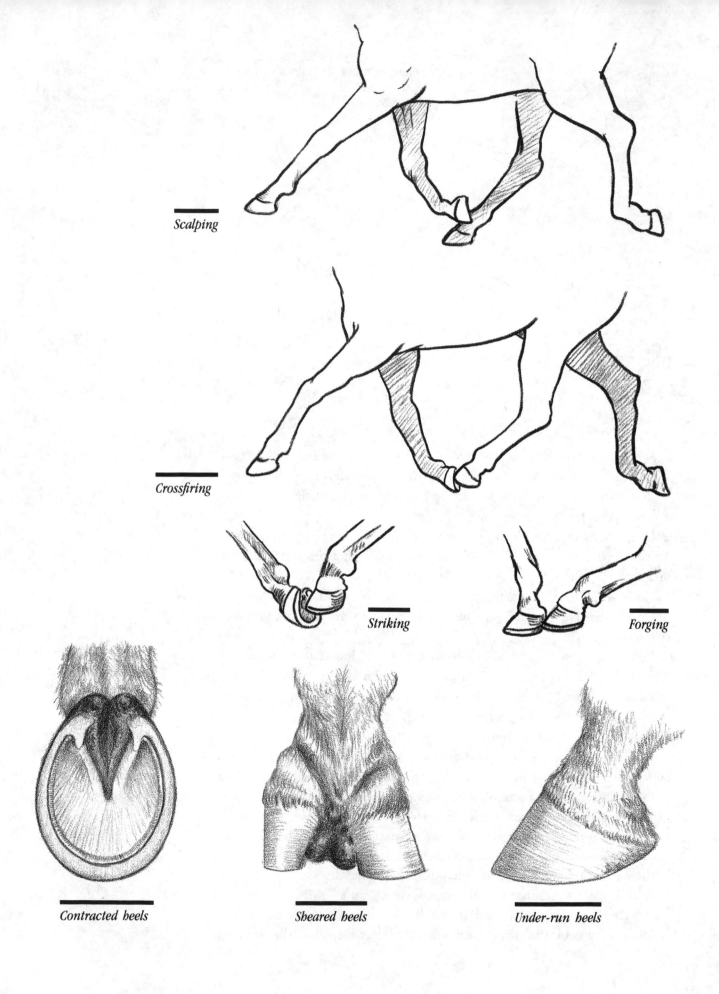

Scalping

Crossfiring

Striking

Forging

Contracted heels

Sheared heels

Under-run heels

in an adult horse remains permanent and may cause lameness or stumbling.

Rings in the wall of the foot may be a normal result of a change in the horse's diet at some time in the past. Blistering of the coronary band may cause a line in the hoof, too. Large lines or rings with a wavy appearance signal a problem in the foot. Laminitis is one of the most common causes of rings in the hoof wall. In this case the rings will diverge, becoming wider at the heel than at the toe.

Your farrier's goal is to balance your horse's foot. The result is a horse with a level foot that lands squarely on both heels. While this sounds simple, it may be difficult to achieve in a horse that has long-standing problems.

You'll need to be patient if your horse has an obvious foot problem. A radical trimming job can make the horse even more lame than before. It may take a year or more to bring the horse's feet gradually toward normal. Some problems, such as a club foot in an adult horse, may not be completely correctable.

Use the time you spend picking out your horse's feet to take a good look at them. Are the inside and outside hoof walls the same length? Do the right and left feet have the same shape, size, and angles? Careful attention to your horse's feet can help you prevent disease from occurring, reduce its effects, and slow the progression of disease.

Soft Soles, Sole Bruises, and Abscesses

Bruising of the sole is a common cause of lameness in the horse. A sole bruise at the angle of the heel is called a corn. Causes of sole bruises include working the horse on hard or uneven ground, overzealous paring of the sole with a hoof knife, and a too-soft or a flat sole. An improperly applied shoe may bruise the foot, as can shoes with heel caulks or toe grabs.

The sole bruise that results from an obvious cause is most easily remedied. A full-bar shoe or shoe with pad are applied to take the pressure off the sore area.

Sole bruising caused by a flat or soft sole can be an ongoing problem. While pads can temporarily relieve the symptoms, they often worsen the problem by further weakening and softening the sole. Moisture accumulates under the pad and the sole has no stimulus for strengthening.

Some veterinarians and farriers will alternate using a shoe with pad and one without at each shoe change. Sole hardeners may be applied to the bottom of the foot during times when it's not protected by a pad. Most hardeners or sole paints consist of a caustic or irritating substance,

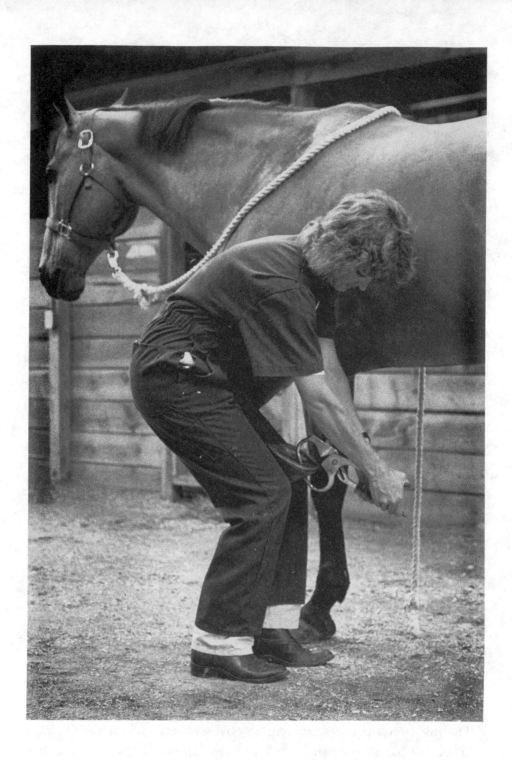

so you should wear gloves and apply the product to the sole of the foot only.

Another cause of foot bruising is a shoe nail driven too close to the sensitive laminae. If the nail penetrates live tissue, an abscess may result. The solution to either problem is to remove the nail.

A foot abscess is more commonly caused by a puncture wound on the bottom of the foot. These infections are excruciatingly painful, and the horse will do anything to prevent putting weight on the leg. The cause of the abscess may be found by a thorough examination of the sole. A nail or wire may sometimes be imbedded there, although the offending cause is often long since gone and you see no sign of a hole.

The cause of the horse's pain is a pocket of pus underneath the hoof wall. You may see an area at the coronary band where the abscess has ruptured onto the surface. There may be a small hole which leaks pus or bloody fluid. In most cases, though, the abscess has not yet opened. You may find that the horse is extremely sensitive when you attempt to pick out its feet. The horse refuses to let you pick up the opposite leg, since it's much too painful to stand on the abscessed foot. Gently lay your hand over the lower pastern area to feel increased warmth in the foot. Compare each foot to the others if you aren't sure.

Your veterinarian can find the sore spot with careful use of hoof testers. This tool looks like a large pair of pliers, and is used to apply pressure to various parts of the foot. Sometimes a radiograph (X ray) is required to find the pocket of infection.

A small hole in the sole is created with a drill or hoof knife so the infection can drain out. Don't rely on drainage at the coronet to resolve the infection; the hole will seal up and the problem will recur. The drainage hole is usually packed with iodine-soaked cotton and the entire foot is wrapped to keep dirt from entering. You may be instructed to soak the foot several times each day, or to apply a poultice to draw out the infection. These measures are as important as any medication you give the horse.

You can prevent an abscess by picking out your horse's feet every day so that you find any punctures when they occur. If you find a nail or wire still embedded in the hoof, pull it out with a pair of pliers. Remember the location of the hole, and save the object to show your veterinarian. You must treat the puncture to prevent an abscess. First, scrub all the dirt off the horse's hoof and sole, which may require immersing the entire foot in a bucket of water. Treatment for punctures will be similar to that for an abscess. Squirt iodine into the hole to prevent infection, and protect the foot from dirt and mud. Show your veterinarian how deeply the object penetrated. The vet may decide that your horse needs antibiotics. Your horse will always need a tetanus booster after a puncture wound.

Navicular Disease

Degeneration of the navicular bone, the small coffin-shaped bone within the hoof, can cause permanent lameness in a severely affected horse. Navicular disease usually affects both front legs, although one may be affected more than the other. The horse with navicular disease will sometimes appear to be lame in just one front leg, but when your veterinarian performs a nerve block, the lameness shifts to the opposite leg.

Use of hoof testers will show that the horse with navicular disease is sore at the heel or in the middle of the frog. The horse tries to land on its toes while trotting and shortens its stride to avoid painful pressure on the navicular bone. The sometimes confusing result can be bruising of the sole at the toe. Your vet will radiograph the navicular area to look for signs of the bone disease.

Navicular disease has been associated with specific hoof problems. While navicular disease is a difficult problem, hope lies in the fact that many of the hoof abnormalities associated with it are correctable by proper trimming and shoeing. When the horse's feet are examined and corrected toward normal form and function, many of his symptoms disappear.

How do you know what's normal, and what's abnormal? You'll need the assistance of your farrier and veterinarian to evaluate your horse. Under-run, contracted, and sheared heels are among the abnormalities associated with navicular disease. These problems can occur in horses without navicular disease as well, so their presence doesn't necessarily mean your horse has that problem.

There have been many different recommendations for corrective shoeing of the horse with navicular disease. Each method meets with success in a certain percentage of horses, but doesn't help others at all. Horses are only helped when their own specific hoof abnormalities are corrected.

Many horses that are sore in the navicular area will improve with just a change in trimming or shoeing. Others need medication as well. Your veterinarian may recommend a combination of shoeing and medications to relieve the symptoms of navicular disease. Although navicular disease cannot be cured, its symptoms can be held at bay, allowing some horses to continue athletic activity.

Laminitis

Laminitis and founder can be devastating diseases for the horse. Laminitis is a disease of the horse's entire system that shows its effects in the animal's feet. Both front legs are usually affected. In severe cases the hind feet may also become sore.

Laminitis is an inflammation of the laminae, the tissues between the hoof wall and the coffin bone. Founder results when those tissues can no longer support the coffin bone, which rotates or sinks out of its normal position. In severe cases, the bone may actually protrude downward through the sole of the foot.

Laminitis can be caused by a dietary indiscretion (overeating of grain or lush pasture), working on hard ground ("road founder"), metritis (a

132

Easy Health Care
For Your Horse

uterine infection in mares), or any severe illness or stress. Black walnut shavings used as bedding can cause severe founder. Certain horses may be prone to laminitis because of hormonal imbalances. The typical horse or pony with hypothyroidism is overweight, has a cresty neck, and tends to develop chronic founder.

In many cases, the syndrome begins with release of endotoxins into the bloodstream. Endotoxins are a part of normal bacteria that live in the horse's gut. When the bacteria die, endotoxins are released. Normal horses do not absorb the toxin, which is swept away with the intestinal contents. In the case of colic, however, intestinal motility slows and the lining of the intestine is damaged. Massive amounts of endotoxins can be released into the horse's system.

Endotoxins alter the blood flow in the foot so that some areas have an increased flow, but circulation within the laminae is decreased. The laminae become inflamed, blood clots form in the vessels, and the tissues die, leaving the coffin bone without support within the hoof.

In mild cases, the horse shifts his weight from one foot to the other. At other times, the pain may be so severe that the horse refuses to walk. A "sawhorse" stance is common; the horse will stretch his front feet forward to take pressure off his sore toes.

Inflammation results in increased heat in the pastern area. In severe cases, you can feel a depression at the coronary band because the coffin bone has sunk out of its normal position.

Acute laminitis is the term used to describe a sudden onset of the disease and the first few days of illness, or as long as the coffin bone is rotating. Horses with chronic laminitis have a recurring problem with flare-ups of acute disease.

In horses with chronic founder, the appearance of the hoof wall and sole reflect the internal damage. The hoof wall develops horizontal lines that are wider at the heel than the toe, and the toe tends to curl upward. You may see a widening of the "white line," the area where the sole meets the hoof wall. The bottom of the sole may become flattened.

A horse with laminitis is an emergency. Firm, supportive ground, such as moist sand or a moderately bedded stall, can make the horse comfortable. Avoid deep, soft footing or hard cement.

Old treatments that are no longer recommended include walking the horse or having the horse stand in cold water. Cold water further constricts the blood vessels in the feet, possibly worsening the condition. Walking the horse injures the already weakened laminae. The best first aid that you can give is to call your veterinarian, then wait for further instructions.

Treatment for laminitis varies tremendously and is still controversial, partly because no single therapy has been proven to work. Your vet might administer a blood vessel dilator, anti-inflammatory medication, and other

Care of Feet
and Hooves

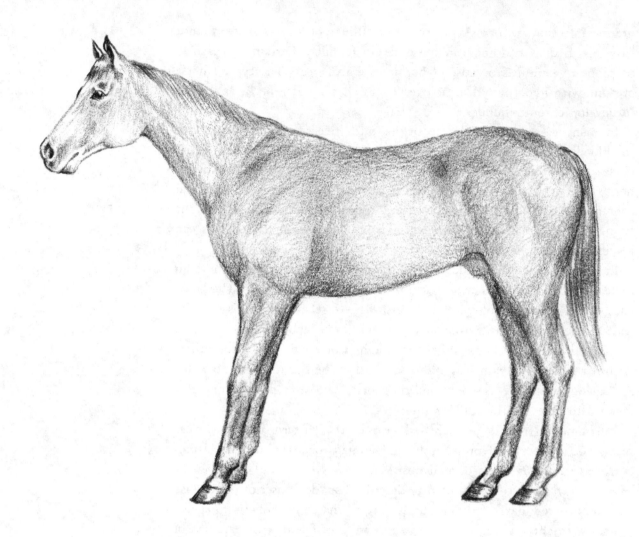

drugs. Anti-endotoxin antiserum is used to fight the effects of endotoxin.

The amount of rotation (measured in degrees of an angle), and sinking (measured in centimeters of drop from normal), that occur are measured on radiographs. Every horse with laminitis is radiographed at least once, and most have several X rays taken to monitor the progress of the disease.

No matter how mild your horse's case of laminitis may seem, at least a month of stall rest is usually required. The laminae must be given time to grow and regain their former strength, or to be replaced by scar tissue. If you let him out for exercise too soon, your horse could suffer a severe setback.

Horses with laminitis can be made much more comfortable with the aid of an experienced farrier and veterinarian. Corrective trimming may be done immediately or postponed until a later date. Shoes are usually not applied during the acute stages of laminitis.

Horses with chronic laminitis often develop infections and abscesses in the feet, since the dying tissues are a haven for bacterial growth. Soaking the feet in hot Epsom salts is sometimes recommended.

Easy Health Care
For Your Horse

If your horse suffers from laminitis or founder, be sure that you fully understand the prognosis for its recovery, what recovery means (a pasture pet, or an athlete), and the cost of its treatment. You must make a commitment to long-term treatment (several months to a year or more), and expect occasional setbacks. Avoid frustration and crushed hopes by adopting a realistic view of your horse's problem at the start.

Most cases of laminitis are preventable. Try to minimize the stress your horse is under, particularly if you are competing hard and traveling most of the time. Have your mare checked after she gives birth to be sure there are no problems with infection or retained afterbirth. Avoid sudden changes in your horse's diet, and keep overweight horses off lush pasture. Ask your veterinarian to examine any horse with colic or digestive upset, and treat overeating as an emergency. Laminitis that results from overeating will occur a day or more after the incident. It is vital that any horse suspected of overeating be treated immediately, rather than waiting to see if symptoms will appear.

Unfortunately, some cases of founder are hopeless despite the best of care. Other horses recover with some degree of disability. The horse with a mild case of laminitis that is treated early in its course stands a good chance of recovery.

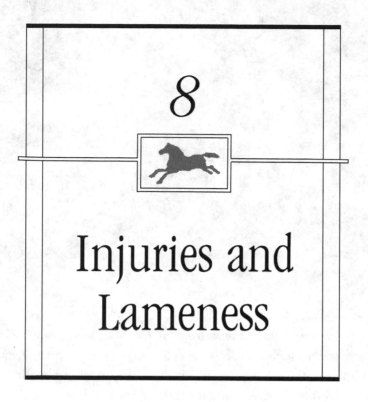

8

Injuries and Lameness

Finding the Problem

The Physical Exam

Whether your horse is sick, injured, or lame, the first thing to do is to perform a physical examination. Take a closer look at your horse while he's healthy, so that you'll know what is normal. Of course you look at your horse every day, but your first aid training starts with a closer look. Don't underestimate these apparently simple tasks. The veterinarian who seems to diagnose your horse's problems with just a quick look has mastered the art of the physical exam.

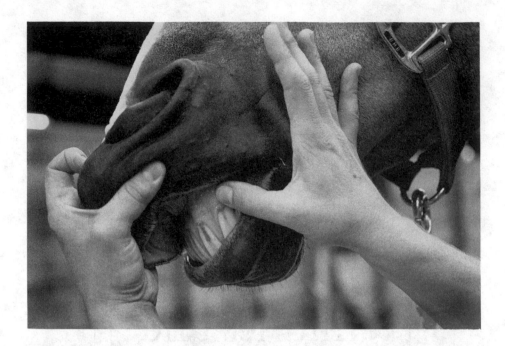

Begin by viewing your horse from a distance. How much time does your horse spend standing, how much time lying down? What is his general conformation? Measure your horse's girth with a weight tape once a month so you will notice weight gain or loss.

Observe your horse's eating and elimination habits. Is your horse a slow eater, or does he gobble up his food? What does the manure look like? Pick up a couple of manure balls and note their consistency, which will vary depending on your horse's diet. Learn what is normal, so that if your horse colics, you can tell whether the manure is dryer or softer than usual.

What is your horse's normal conformation? Note any old splints, lumps or bumps, and their sizes. Run your hands over all four legs, getting used to the natural form of your horse's body. When you pick out the feet, notice the normal texture and clean odor.

Look carefully at your horse's head. Examine the ears, nostrils, and eyes. Is there normally some discharge from the eyes on dusty days? How much? Lift your horse's lip and notice the moist, pink gums. Their color can become pale or bluish with blood loss, colic, or shock.

Pressing your finger against the gum leaves a white spot that fills back with pink within a second or two. The capillary refill time is a measure of the vigor of the horse's circulation. A horse that is dehydrated or in shock will have a delayed refill time because its circulation is compromised.

What is your horse's normal breathing pattern? You'll need a watch with a second hand to count the respiratory rate. Watch the horse's flank and count the movements in one minute. A resting horse will breathe about eight to twenty times per minute, while the rate goes up to sixty

Easy Health Care
For Your Horse

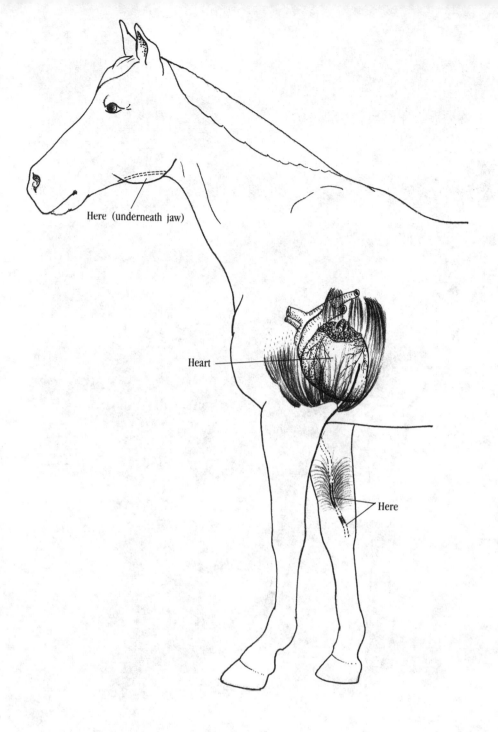

Here (underneath jaw)

Heart

Here

or more with strenuous exercise. Pain, colic, and respiratory infections can cause an increase in the respiratory rate.

You can take your horse's pulse in several places; try them all and use the one that is easiest for you. To feel the pulse, place your fingertips along the jawbone, inside the knee, under the tail, or on the outside of the rear cannon bone.

You are feeling for the pulse of blood through your horse's arteries. Locate the artery by sliding your fingertips (not your thumb which has its own pulse) over the area until you find the thin, cordlike vessel. If

139

Injuries and
Lameness

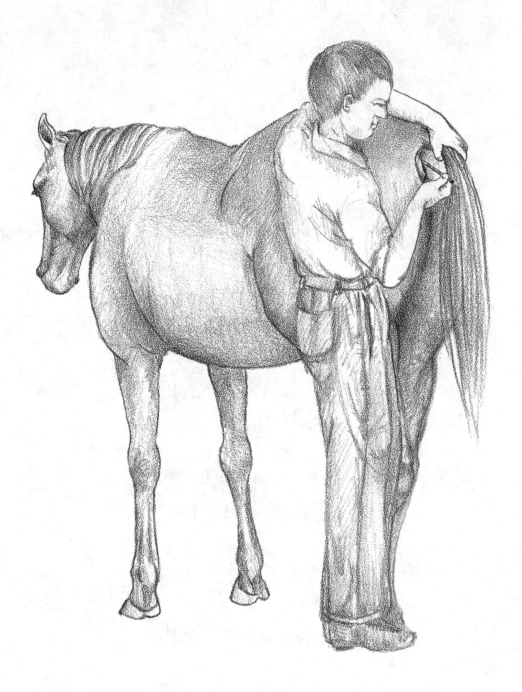

you have difficulty feeling the pulse, vary the amount of pressure over the vessel.

You can listen to the heart with a stethoscope or feel the heart rate directly on the horse's left side. Place your stethoscope or the palm of your hand just behind the horse's elbow. You may have to push up and inward to reach behind the elbow of a horse with a large forearm.

Count the number of beats in fifteen seconds and multiply that by four to get the pulse rate. A horse's pulse rate will range from thirty-two to forty per minute while resting to over one hundred per minute with

Easy Health Care
For Your Horse

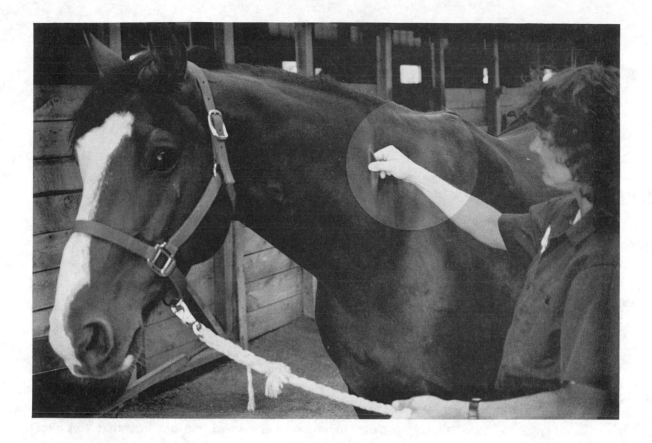

exercise. Each horse has a different resting pulse rate, and knowing your horse's rate will help you evaluate changes. Pain, fear, or blood loss will all cause an increase in the pulse rate.

Like the pulse, body temperature varies with each horse. Take your horse's temperature for several days in a row. Normal temperatures range from 98 to 101°F.

You can use a special horse thermometer or a human rectal thermometer. Shake down the mercury, lubricate the tip, and insert it a couple of inches into your horse's rectum. Leave it there for two or three minutes, then read the mercury level.

If the thermometer is misplaced, it is probably on the ground, not lost inside your horse. Attach a string to the thermometer, and an alligator clip or clothespin to the end of the string. Attach that end to your horse's tail so your thermometer doesn't break if it falls out.

There are several ways that you can tell whether your horse is dehydrated. Each sign must be compared to that particular horse's normal situation. First, look at the gums. Normally they are moist; they become dry and sticky in the dehydrated horse. Next, take a small pinch of skin on the horse's neck and notice how long it takes to fall flat again. The dehydrated horse's skin will "tent" and remain in place for several seconds. With severe dehydration, the horse's eyes appear sunken.

Practice your physical exam once a week. Soon it will take only a few minutes to give your horse a thorough going-over. If accidents or illness strike, you'll be calm and ready to evaluate the problem. Instead of being able to little more than say, "he isn't acting right," you will have specific information that can help you decide what to do.

Emergency First Aid: Deciding What to Do

First aid involves both an evaluation of a problem and the immediate assistance that you provide for your horse. We'll cover what to do in specific situations in the following sections. No matter what the problem is, though, your immediate first aid step is the same. When you first realize that your horse is in trouble, remain calm and think clearly. Put a halter and lead rope on your horse and keep him calm, too, to prevent further injury. Then survey the situation and decide what to do next.

Don't try to move an injured horse until you are sure that you won't aggravate the injury. Send someone for help while you stay with the horse. Keep your own safety in mind above all else. Sometimes there is no way you can restrain such a big animal, and the horse might injure you because of fright or pain. If you can't hold the horse, leave him alone until help arrives.

There are a few cases where slow walking is necessary to prevent further injury to your horse. Walk the horse during a painful colic episode or if a severe case of itchy hives is causing him to mutilate himself with scratching.

Immediate life-threatening situations include bleeding and broken bones. If you see an obvious fracture, if there is protruding bone, a strange angle in the leg, or the horse won't put any weight on the leg, don't move the horse until help arrives.

Do you see spurting blood, or is there bleeding that won't stop? Although all cuts and scrapes bleed a little, you must be concerned about severe blood loss. Apply firm, direct pressure to the bleeding area and leave it on to help stop the flow. Anything you have handy can be used as a pressure wrap: gauze squares, a diaper, or even a T-shirt or rag in an emergency. Secure your padding with gauze roll or tape. If blood soaks through your wrap, just apply more bandage material on top; removing what's already there will disturb the clot.

If there is not an obvious injury, conduct a thorough physical exam. Even if one injury demands your immediate attention, you'll still need to complete your exam so you don't overlook other, less severe problems.

Easy Health Care
For Your Horse

There may be times when your horse just "isn't doing well." Rather than wait to see what happens, carefully go through your physical exam. You may find that your horse is coming down with a respiratory infection or has a mild case of colic or any one of many other problems. Your exam will help you focus on the problem and catch it early.

After you do your physical examination, call your veterinarian. The vet will usually want to look at your horse before giving advice over the phone, especially if you are not a regular client. Still, if you've done a thorough physical, your vet is less likely to say, "I can't give you advice without looking at the horse," and you'll be more likely to call, knowing that the vet won't come out unless you both know it's necessary. As you gain experience, you will be able to handle small problems yourself.

Your First Aid Kit

Along with having a first aid kit ready for an emergency, you must know what to use and how to use it in specific situations. Ask your veterinarian to help you stock your first aid kit. You may need more than is listed here. Promptly restock used items, and always ask your veterinarian whenever you aren't sure what to do in an emergency.

Basic supplies include the following:

Halter and lead rope	Syringe (without needle, for
Thermometer	flushing)
Needle-nose pliers with wire	Bucket
cutters	Antibacterial ointment
Twitch	Antibacterial powder
Hoof pick and hoof knife	Nonadherent wound pads
Clippers	Disposable diaper or cotton roll
Hemostats or tweezers	Ace bandage or Vetrap
Gauze squares	2-inch wide white tape
Iodine soap	3-inch elastic tape
Tamed iodine solution	3-inch gauze roll
Sterile saline	Duct tape
Alcohol	Suture-removal scissors
	Bandage scissors

What are you going to do with all this? As you read this and the next chapter, you'll gather information for specific problems. In general, though, here's how you will use the different parts of your kit.

When you notice that your horse is sick or injured, you will have to put a halter and lead rope on him. That way you have control of the horse and can perform a complete physical exam, including taking his temperature.

Needle-nose pliers with wire cutters will untangle fence wire or pull a nail from your horse's foot. Use your hoof pick and hoof knife to examine your horse's feet. You might need the twitch to restrain the horse while you examine an injury. Clippers remove hair that blocks your view of a wound.

Hemostats or tweezers help remove splinters. Use the gauze squares to clean a wound with iodine soap or solution. Your bucket will be filled with warm water to help your clean-up effort, or with ice water to cool a sprain or strain.

Fill the syringe with sterile saline to flush your horse's eyes. To flush a puncture wound, fill the syringe with water, sterile saline, or tamed iodine solution (diluted 1:10 with water or saline). Saline is 0.9 percent sodium chloride (salt), and is better than plain water for flushing wounds.

Apply antibacterial ointment to a scrape that tends to become dry. Use the powder, instead, if the wound is weepy or moist. Do not apply either if the veterinarian is coming, since the medication may not be desirable if stitches are needed; besides, the vet will remove any medication that you apply to get a better look at the wound. (If you are concerned that a wound might dry out or needs protection while you wait for a veterinarian, cover it with a clean, moistened cloth or a light wrap.)

The nonadherent dressing (Telfa), gauze roll, and other bandage materials are used for different types of wraps (see "Bandages," below). You will need bandage scissors to cut wrap material and to remove the wrap. Use suture scissors if your vet has you remove stitches.

Duct tape is essential for quick and dirty repairs of tack or equipment, for keeping a wrap on the bottom of your horse's foot, and for countless other little mishaps. Do not apply duct tape to your horse's skin, though, since it is too stiff. An elastic tape is preferable on the skin.

Scrapes and Cuts

Early morning feeding is usually a peaceful time. Fresh air and the sound of nickering horses help open your sleepy eyes. One morning, though, you don't hear the nickering, and your horse doesn't come running in from the pasture as usual. A quick look around reveals your horse standing under a group of trees with a large flap of skin dangling from its leg. Your horse couldn't have chosen a less convenient time to get into trouble.

This story sounds familiar to many horse owners. Scrapes and cuts are the most common injuries that you will encounter. While you can't protect your horse from every possible injury, you can frequently prevent those accidents from turning into disasters.

First Aid

Fortunately, most cuts and scrapes aren't life-or-death situations that require immediate action. You have time to gather your thoughts and your first aid kit, then proceed to examine the wound carefully. Horses have a lot of blood, and any cut will usually bleed a little.

Smaller vessels usually stop bleeding on their own. Bleeding that won't stop by itself after a few minutes requires action on your part. If an artery is cut, you will see a spurt of blood with each heart beat. Injuries to larger veins, on the other hand, will ooze continuously.

A clean cloth or gauze sponge held onto the bleeding area will stop the flow. Apply firm, continuous pressure for several minutes rather than dabbing or wiping at the area. If the bleeding resumes when you release your pressure, use an elastic wrap or gauze roll to hold the cloth in place. Always call the veterinarian if you can't get bleeding to stop within several minutes.

Avoid using tourniquets; they can cause permanent damage since they totally block any blood flow to the area below the band. If you cannot get the bleeding to stop, you probably have not left the wrap on long enough for a clot to form or haven't applied pressure firmly enough.

Assuming your horse isn't bleeding severely, you're ready to clean the wound and take a closer look. Don't worry about what you're going to put on the wound until you clean off everything—your Magic Purple Potion won't do a bit of good when it's sprayed over dirt and scabs.

What should you use to clean a wound? Many antiseptics are irritating when used improperly, so if you aren't sure, don't use them. Your goal is to wash out dirt, debris, and bacteria, not to put something on the wound that will "neutralize" the dirt. Use scissors or clippers to remove hair around wounds, and clean, warm water to remove dirt and debris.

If you feel that you must use something special to clean the wound, your best choices are either tamed iodine solution (not tincture of iodine; see chapter 4) diluted 1:10 with water; iodine soap (be sure to rinse well); or normal saline, which is 0.9 percent sodium chloride (obtain one-liter bottles from your vet, or use the saline that is sold for rinsing soft contact lenses). Use a washcloth, gauze sponges, or paper towels to remove hair, dirt, and caked-on blood. Continue until you see only clean, pink flesh.

You'll be lucky if you find your horse immediately after an injury occurs, while the wound is still clean. The usual course is to discover the injury when it is already several hours old, caked with dirt and blood. The wound is swollen, painful, and difficult to clean. The easiest way to deal with this type of wound is simply to hold a running hose on it for fifteen minutes or so. The cool water will soothe the area, decrease swelling, and soften and loosen the dirt. You can then begin to clean the area gently with your cloth or gauze sponges.

Even if the cut appears small, proceed with your cleansing until you can see the all the edges of the cut and only pink flesh. Gently spread the cut open to see how deep it is. Close examination of an apparently minor wound may reveal a deep puncture or cut. You'll want to find out immediately, rather than after infection has set in.

Don't worry if your washing causes the wound to begin to bleed again. This is normal, and unless it is excessive, you can finish your job before applying a wrap to stop the bleeding.

Remove hair around the wound with clippers so you can see it better and so hairs won't irritate the injury. If you don't have clippers, use blunt-tipped scissors to cut off longer hairs at the wound edges. Since matted hair will resist your clipping efforts, soften and moisten the area with warm water so your clippers will be effective, or alternate clipping and washing to remove all the dirt and hair gradually.

Difficulty with restraining your horse for an exam or treatment can become a major obstacle to his recovery. The first step in overcoming this problem is to work on your horse before he's injured, especially if he is reluctant to have you handle certain parts of his body. Ask your trainer to help you with problem areas.

Some horses simply need to be restrained in cross-ties to stop their fidgeting. It's safer, though, to have someone hold your horse while you work. The person should stand on the same side of the horse that you are working on, and should devote all attention to the horse—not to what you are doing. Sometimes a light "neck twitch" provides just enough restraint; have your handler grab a fold of skin on the neck and pinch lightly.

Even the well-trained horse will resist having a painful area touched. You must consider that some restraint will be necessary for your own safety and so you can get the job done. Use a nose twitch or a lip chain to divert his attention. These are humane methods of restraint when used properly; have your trainer show you how.

When to Call the Vet

Now that you've cleaned the wound and can see the entire injury, you must decide whether to treat it yourself or to call a veterinarian. Wounds in certain areas should always be evaluated by a veterinarian, no matter how small or minor they may seem at first. Any cut that is over a joint, into a tendon, or below the pastern can cause long-term trouble, so it should always be examined by a veterinarian:

Easy Health Care
For Your Horse

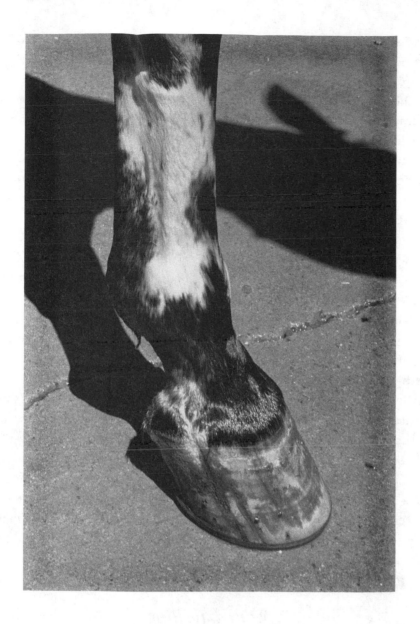

If bacteria enter a joint, the resulting infection may mean months of treatment and sometimes permanent lameness. Postponing treatment for even a day can mean the difference between a quick recovery and long-term problems.

Tendon injuries often heal poorly. Portions of the tendons on the lower legs are surrounded by a fluid-lined sheath, which can become infected. An infected tendon sheath can drain continuously, preventing healing.

Cuts at the heel area tend to spread open with each step the horse takes, preventing healing for long periods of time.

Any coronary band injury can cause permanent changes in growth of the hoof wall. These need veterinary attention immediately.

Injuries to other areas may need sutures (stitches). How do you know whether a cut needs sutures? Just about any cut will heal better if it stays clean and its edges are held together with sutures. Of course, many cuts heal without stitches, but the healing is delayed and the potential for scar formation is much greater. If you can see pink flesh under a cut, then it probably needs stitches.

Injuries that can't be sutured include scrapes, deep cuts into the muscle, and old injuries. While it's obvious that scrapes cannot be sutured, you may wonder why vets don't suture large cuts in the horse's muscle. Unfortunately, muscle tissue doesn't hold stitches well. Even a beautiful surgical repair may fill with fluid after several days, causing the suture knots to fail.

An injury that is over six to eight hours old also will hold stitches poorly. Often the swelling is so severe that the skin edges cannot be brought together. Older cuts tend to become infected, too. Closing the skin over an infected area will only lead to worse infection. In some cases, though, the dead and infected tissues can be trimmed away, creating a "fresh" cut that can then be sutured.

Allow your vet to make the decision about whether large cuts should be sutured rather than trying to decide yourself. Sometimes large wounds are sutured even though it's likely that the stitches will eventually fail—at least there is a temporary covering over the wound.

Whether or not you call your veterinarian, be sure that your horse has had a recent tetanus vaccination. Most veterinarians will give a tetanus booster to any injured horse unless one was given in the past few months, in spite of the usual recommendation of yearly tetanus boosters for uninjured horses.

Wound Healing

What can you do to help your horse's wound heal quickly? Remember that clean tissues heal best. Before you ask which powder, spray, or ointment is best for your horse's cut, recall that a wound that stays clean heals much faster than one that simply has something sprayed on each day.

This means you must go back to the cleansing step every day. Gently soak off dirt and scabs with warm water until you can see pink, clean wound edges, after which you might apply ointment to a scrape that tends to dry out, or a spray or powder to the wound that oozes serum. (See chapter 4.)

There is no single wound treatment that is best for all injuries. Be sure to read the label and ask your veterinarian if you aren't sure. Some products are ideal in one situation but disastrous in another.

Easy Health Care
For Your Horse

For example, scarlet oil is a preparation used on deep injuries in the muscle. Its slightly irritating effect helps the defect to close in quickly. When used below the knee or hock, though, scarlet oil can delay healing or cause growth of proud flesh (excess scar tissue).

Which wounds should be kept under wraps? Cuts on the horse's legs often require a support wrap to minimize swelling. Other injuries quickly become dirty or fly-infested if left open. But healing is fastest on some wounds if they are left open. Certain areas just can't hold a wrap (the shoulder, for example). The choice will depend on the extent of the injury, its location, and on the horse. (See "Bandages," below.)

Normal wounds heal by the gradual growth of tissue over the injured area. This flat bed of granulation tissue is then slowly covered by normal skin and hair. The healing system can go awry, though, and granulation tissue can grow beyond its bounds. The resulting cauliflower-like growth called proud flesh prohibits normal skin and hair from covering the area.

Your veterinarian calls this excess tissue growth *exuberant granulation tissue*. Proud flesh occurs on the legs from the knee or hock downward, in areas with excess movement and tight skin. Irritating medications, dirt, infection, or a bandage that is too tight aggravate the growth. Proud flesh can be prevented by immobilizing the area and keeping the wound clean and wrapped.

Call your vet as soon as you notice the beginning of proud flesh, since it is much easier to control early on. You might use a slightly caustic wound dressing that eats away at the growth, but always use caustic medications only with your veterinarian's supervision to avoid burning the horse's normal tissues. Sometimes the only solution is for your veterinarian to surgically shave off the excess tissue, rewrap the injury, allow for a little more healing, and then repeat the process.

Five Basic Rules for Wounds

One: Apply pressure to bleeding wounds. Call the vet if you can't stop the bleeding within several minutes.

Two: Clean everything *off* before you put anything *on.*

Three: Wounds over a joint, into a tendon, near the heels, or on the coronary band should *always* receive veterinary attention.

Four: Be sure that your horse has had a recent tetanus vaccination.

Five: Healing is best with a clean wound. The best medication to apply after cleansing depends on many factors, including the wound type and location. Do *not* use the same product for every injury.

Injuries and
Lameness

Bandages

All horse owners must learn how to apply leg wraps. No matter how much you read, you still need lots of practice before you can apply a wrap that stays up and does its job. Use the guidelines here to get started, then ask someone experienced for help the first time you try to apply a wrap.

Bandage Materials

There are an infinite number of bandage materials, but they all fall into a few categories. Have enough of each type to wrap all four legs if necessary; buy washable materials rather than disposable ones if possible.

Wound protection: Use a nonadherent dressing, such as a Telfa pad, or gauze squares.

Plastic wrap: Use plastic food wrap, or a plastic bag cut into a flat piece, for sweats and poultices.

Paddings: Leg cottons or quilts, disposable or nondisposable diapers, roll cotton, or U.S. Army Field Bandages can be used for padding. Use disposable diapers with the plastic side toward the horse for a sweat, or with the dry side toward the horse for a padded wrap.

Roll bandage: Brown or white roll gauze in three- or four-inch widths holds the padding in place, and comes in stretch and nonstretch varieties. Use flannel wraps for a washable alternative.

Stretch wrap: Ace bandage or Vetrap in three- or four-inch widths are used to increase a wrap's pressure and hold the wrap firmly in place. Vetrap is self-adhering but still needs some tape to hold the end down.

Elastic tape: Elasticon or similar tape is used for securing the top and bottom of the wrap. It can be applied to the leg and on skin, but stretching too tightly cuts off circulation.

Nonelastic tape: Use duct tape to secure bandage material to the hoof and foot only; do not use it on the leg. Electrician's tape or white tape can be used to secure the outer layer of the bandage, but it is not the best choice for the horse's skin. Beware of applying it too tightly.

Types of Wraps and Bandages

Why would you apply a wrap to your horse's legs? Each situation requires a different type of wrap, boot, or bandage. Know the differences between wraps and use each where it is needed. After you decide what you want the wrap to accomplish, then the choice is easier.

Apply wraps or boots to protect a horse's legs from injury during rest or exercise. Apply a bandage over an open wound to protect it from dirt and flies. Wrap over a cut that has been stitched to prevent the stitches from being disturbed and to reduce swelling. Also, wrap a lower leg after any sprain, strain, or wound that causes the leg to swell.

Stable or standing bandages are left on the horse while the animal is not being worked. These bandages come in a variety of materials: flannel, cotton, wool, and quilted. Shipping boots or leg wraps are put on the horse to protect its legs during trailering. While these wraps protect the leg from minor scrapes or cuts, they don't provide major support to the leg. At best, the wrap prevents filling (swelling) that occurs when the horse must stand in one position for a long time.

Stable bandages, standing bandages, and shipping boots all cover the legs from below the knee or hock down to the pastern or coronet. You can use one type of bandage or wrap to serve several purposes. Be aware that horses don't need to have all four legs wrapped every night. Constant wrapping can even damage the legs by decreasing circulation.

Bandages or boots are applied to protect the legs during work, too. This category includes splint boots (worn on the front legs to protect the splint bone and ankle), run-down patches (worn on racehorse's ankles), skid boots (for the back legs of reining horses), bell boots (to protect the coronary band), and exercise bandages (polo wraps, track bandages).

As with standing bandages, exercise wraps protect the leg from cuts or scrapes but they do not provide much support. Since boots can rub or irritate the leg, consider a light wrap underneath the boot (just one layer of an elastic bandage) to protect the leg from rubbing.

Other wraps are applied to prevent or reduce swelling. Dry padded wraps are applied to the legs of a horse that tends to "stock up" (develop swelling in all four legs after standing for several hours). Leg cottons or quilts are put on the leg and held in place with an elastic bandage or roll gauze and electrician's tape. (Another way to reduce minor swelling is to exercise the horse lightly or turn it out, since standing in a stall aggravates the problem.)

Make a sweat wrap to reduce swelling by applying a liquid or ointment to the leg (see chapter 4), then covering the leg with a piece of plastic film. A gauze roll or elastic bandage holds the wrap in place.

Wet or cold wraps reduce swelling after exercise or reduce inflammation after an acute injury. You can make an ice boot with a plastic garbage bag (put your horse's foot in the bag, fill with ice, tape in place), or buy a ready-made one.

Make a cold wrap by soaking bandages in ice water, applying them to the leg, then keeping the wraps cold and wet by pouring more ice water on them. A cool wrap can be made by applying bandage material to the

Injuries and
Lameness

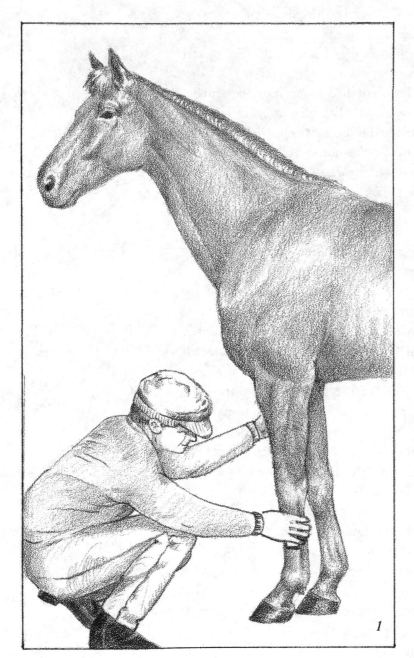

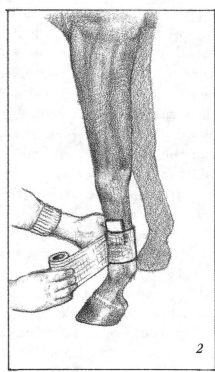

leg and soaking the wrap with rubbing alcohol (this technique does not apply enough cold to treat an injury, but is fine to reduce minor swelling or for cooling out after exercise).

Apply wraps or bandages to an injury (a wound, sprain, or strain) to provide protection and support and to prevent swelling. Several layers are needed. First, apply a nonadherent dressing over any wound that might be present. The dressing is held in place with roll gauze or a short piece of tape.

Apply padding next. Whether or not you need padding is determined by the amount of swelling and how much pressure and support you want

Easy Health Care
For Your Horse

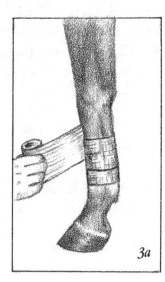
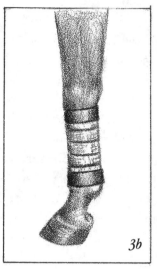
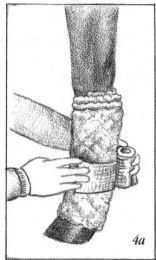
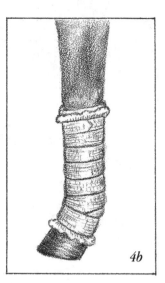

3a *3b* *4a* *4b*

to create. Alternate layers of padding and gauze roll to provide greater support. Use roll cotton, quilts, or a diaper, held in place with more roll gauze.

Use an elastic bandage to hold everything in place and to apply further pressure. Leave the padding protruding from the top and bottom of the wrap. Elastic tape or white tape is applied last, at the top and bottom of the wrap, to prevent dirt from getting under the bandage. Wraps that extend to the foot can be secured there with duct tape.

How to Apply a Wrap

No matter what type of wrap you apply, follow certain guidelines every time. Apply medication and then gauze squares or a nonadherent dressing over a wound. (See chapter 4 for a discussion of wound dressings.) Then decide whether or not you need padding, as discussed above. If no padding is used, the next layer is roll gauze or elastic bandage.

If you use padding, cut it into a rectangle that is just wide enough to encircle the leg once. (If that is not thick enough, alternate layers of padding and gauze roll until you achieve the desired thickness). The length of the rectangle depends on the area you want to cover.

A short piece of padding can be used if you are wrapping only the pastern or only the knees. For most lower leg injuries, though, your padding should extend from just below the knee or hock down to the coronary band. While exercise bandages can end at the ankle, therapeutic bandages should extend all the way down to the coronary band to prevent swelling of the lower leg.

With your gauze roll or elastic bandage, start over the injured area or the center of the wrap, spiraling the wrap material around the leg. Work your way up and then down the leg. Apply wrap material with even pressure, overlapping half the previous section with each turn around the leg. The wrap material should lie flat without bunching or curling. Use a figure-of-eight pattern around the knee, hock, and foot (see below).

The wrap material must be applied snugly enough to create light pressure on the leg and not fall off or bunch up. At the same time, pressure must be even and not too tight to avoid cutting off circulation or creating rub sores. The amount of pressure you can apply to any wrap depends on how much padding you have. An elastic wrap material can be pulled snugly over a thick layer of roll cotton on the leg. Allow the padding to protrude from the top and bottom of the wrap.

Applying the correct amount of pressure takes practice. When finished with a wrap, you should just be able to slide one or two fingers under it; any more or less means the wrap is too loose or too tight. One final step: secure the top and bottom of each wrap with elastic tape; half the tape should be on the horse's hair, half on the wrap.

Swelling above or below the wrap signals that it is too tight. Make a vertical snip with your scissors at the top of the wrap, extending about a half-inch downward, to relieve a moderately tight bandage. Otherwise, replace the entire wrap.

Many horse owners think it essential to wrap each leg in a particular direction—starting on the inside of the leg, then wrapping toward the front, so the wrap winds from front to back on the outside of the leg. In theory, the tendons at the back at the leg thus lie in their normal positions on the leg. However, if you don't wrap the leg too tightly in the first place, there should be no problem with either direction of wrapping.

How often should you change a wrap? The answer depends on the reason for applying the wrap as well as on how well the wrap stays put. "Weepy" wounds will require daily bandage changes. A wrap that bunches up or loosens needs changing, too. Sweat wraps should be changed every twelve to twenty-four hours. Some injuries can get by with a wrap change every two to three days. A bandage over a simple cut that was sutured can stay on longer, if it's in good shape. Ask your vet if you aren't sure.

A wound must be thoroughly cleaned each time you change the wrap. Use warm water and iodine soap, rinse thoroughly, then dry the area with a towel before you apply medication and the wrap. Do the same cleansing when you change a sweat wrap.

Any time your horse has a leg injury, remember also to wrap the leg opposite the injury (use a dry support wrap with light padding). The opposite leg also needs support, since it will take more stress while the injured leg is resting.

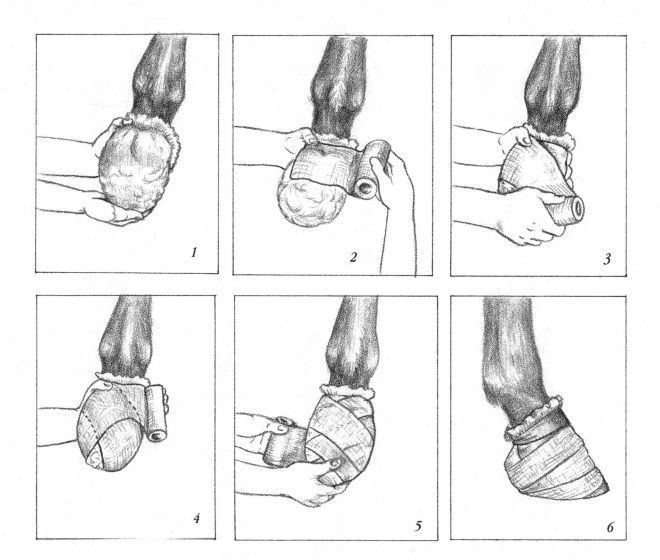

Some horses won't leave a wrap alone. You can apply foul-tasting substances (Tabasco or commercial products) to the wrap itself, or use a neck brace to prevent the horse from reaching its legs.

There are tricks you can use to keep a wrap in place on the angles of your horse's legs. All are based on a figure-of-eight pattern that creates an X across or around areas that bend or protrude.

The foot or lower pastern are bandaged with similar techniques. Clean any wound thoroughly before you start, and scrub all dirt off the hoof wall and sole. Start your wrap with a turn of your material around the pastern. Once you have the wrap started, carry it around and under the bulbs of the heels, keeping firm pressure as you go.

Prevent the wrap material from riding up onto the pastern by hooking it under the heel bulbs or around the entire foot with each pass. Use a figure-of-eight pattern and gradually cover the entire affected area. Don't wrap too high toward the ankle or else the wrap will curl downward. If

Injuries and
Lameness

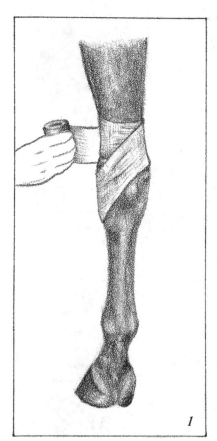
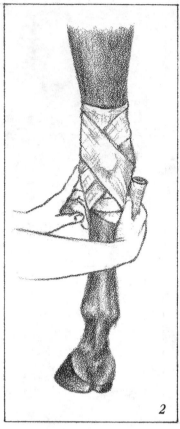
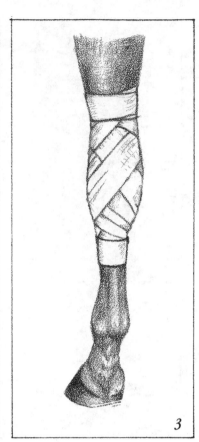

you must extend the wrap up past the ankle, do figures of eight around
that joint too.

Seal the top of the wrap from invading dirt with a piece of elastic
tape. The bottom of a foot wrap will stay on much longer if you build
it up with duct tape. Precut several pieces of duct tape about eight inches
long, pick up the foot, and lay them in a line across the bottom of the
sole so they all extend up the hoof wall an inch or so. Then let the foot
down and encircle the ends of your strips with a piece of tape that goes
all the way around the lower part of the hoof.

Wrapping the fetlock (ankle) is easier if you bring the wrap from the
area a few inches above the ankle all the way down to the foot. Start
above the ankle, making normal turns of the wrap around the leg. When
you reach the ankle, figure-of-eight the wrap around the joint, then take
a couple of turns around the pastern. Finally, secure the wrap at its base
by pulling it down under the bulbs of the heels (as described for the foot
wrap above). Apply elastic tape to the top and bottom of the wrap.

With a little practice, the knee is not difficult to wrap. Start three
inches above the joint and end several inches below. Use figures of eight
across the front and back of the joint. Try to leave the accessory carpal
bone (the bone that protrudes at the back of the knee) exposed between

Easy Health Care
For Your Horse

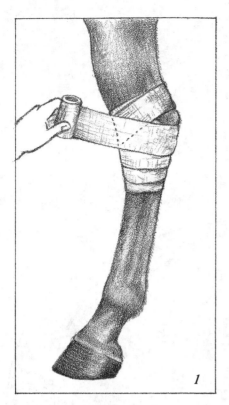
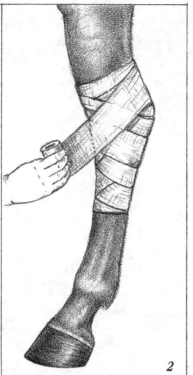
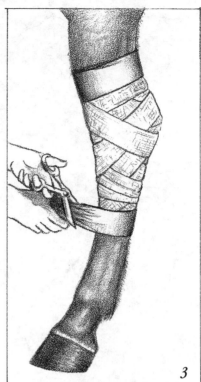

1   *2*   *3*

the holes in your eights, since pressure there could create a sore. Cover the entire wrap with elastic tape for extra security.

You may need to extend a knee or hock wrap all the way down to the coronary band if the injury causes the entire leg to swell. It's easier first to apply one wrap to the joint, then start a second wrap from below the joint down to the foot. Use a light layer of padding on the entire leg.

The hock is wrapped in a similar way. Unless the point of the hock needs to be included in the wrap, leave it out. Carry your wrap material around the hock in a figure of eight, leaving the point of the hock sticking out through a hole in the eight. Finish off with elastic tape.

Another option for wrapping the hock is to protect the Achilles tendon (the tendon above and at the back of the hock) by placing an entire flannel or gauze roll on either side of the tendon. Then, as you pass your wrap material in a figure of eight around the hock, you are not placing direct pressure on that tendon.

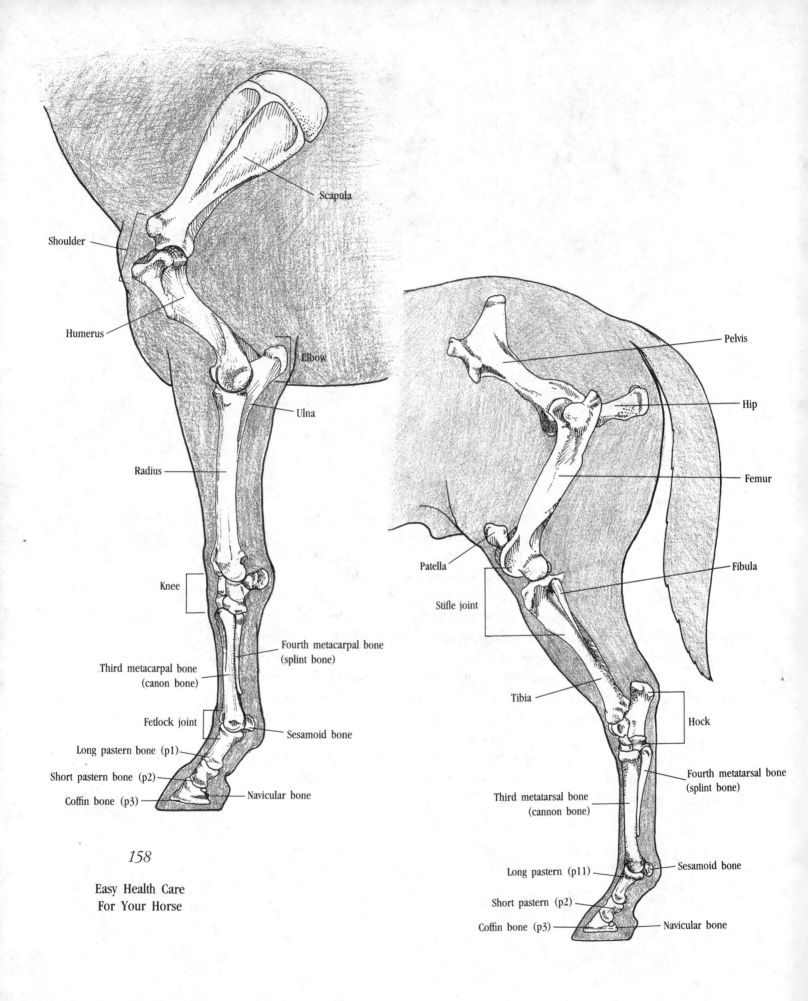

Scapula

Shoulder

Humerus

Elbow

Ulna

Radius

Knee

Third metacarpal bone
(canon bone)

Fourth metacarpal bone
(splint bone)

Fetlock joint

Sesamoid bone

Long pastern bone (p1)

Short pastern bone (p2)

Coffin bone (p3)

Navicular bone

Pelvis

Hip

Femur

Fibula

Patella

Stifle joint

Tibia

Hock

Fourth metatarsal bone
(splint bone)

Third metatarsal bone
(cannon bone)

Long pastern (p11)

Sesamoid bone

Short pastern (p2)

Coffin bone (p3)

Navicular bone

Lameness

It is a rare owner or rider who has never seen a horse become lame. Usually the problem is minor or occurs gradually, giving you plenty of time to get help and advice. But sprains and strains, broken bones, foot abscesses, or founder can result in a horse's sudden reluctance to walk or, just as bad, a leg left dangling helplessly.

The study of legs and lameness could consume a large amount of your time. As a start, learn the anatomy of your horse's legs. Study the diagrams in this chapter first, then see whether you can identify the different structures on your horse. This chapter will help you learn how to locate the source of your horse's lameness and will describe first aid for leg injuries. You'll also be introduced to the most common sources of lameness in the horse.

There are so many different causes of lameness in horses, with so many different treatments, that we cannot discuss them all in detail here. Treatments are constantly being improved, and every horse is treated differently depending on the circumstances. The subjects of rehabilitation and training after an injury would fill an entire book. For detailed information on legs and lameness, consult the classic book, *Adams' Lameness in Horses.* (It and other sources of information are included in the appendix.)

Sudden and Severe Lameness

Causes and First Aid

Finding your horse unable to walk or standing on three legs can be a frightening experience. What you do during those first few hours can make a big difference in how your horse recovers.

Don't wait for an injury to occur to start thinking about your horse's legs. Spend time each day not only looking, but also carefully palpating (feeling) all the structures that make up the legs. Have your veterinarian or trainer help you identify the major muscles, tendons, ligaments, and joints.

Palpate each structure individually so you know what it normally feels like. After an injury, you will palpate the leg in the same way, feeling for heat and swelling or searching for a sore area. Use your fingertips to find soreness, swelling or bumps and the back of your hand to feel for heat. Use gentle, firm pressure to find any painful areas. If your horse flinches or draws the leg away, compare his reaction on the opposite leg to be sure he's really sore there and not just reacting normally.

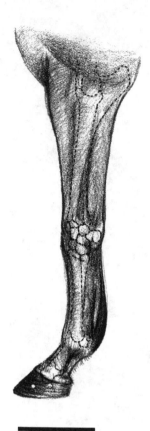

Bowed tendon

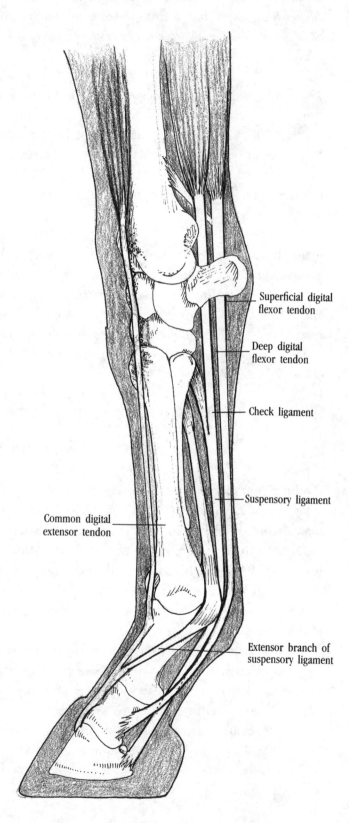

Superficial digital
flexor tendon

Deep digital
flexor tendon

Check ligament

Suspensory ligament

Common digital
extensor tendon

Extensor branch of
suspensory ligament

**Easy Health Care
For Your Horse**

Finding the Cause

A horse that suddenly becomes lame needs attention quickly. How can you tell what the problem is? What first aid can you provide?

Sudden lameness can result from a wide variety of problems. If you see a severely lame horse, take a closer look. Is one leg obviously affected, or is the horse just reluctant to walk at all? Are any obvious swellings present? Did you see an accident happen, or was the horse found lame in its stall or pasture? The answers to these questions will help you narrow down the problem.

Any horse that becomes suddenly lame must be seen by a veterinarian. If you can narrow down the problem area, then your call to the veterinarian might result in your receiving specific instructions on first aid measures that will help the horse while you wait.

Sprains and Strains

A strain is the stretch or tear of a muscle or tendon. Tendons are fibrous bands that attach muscle to bone. As a rule, tendon injuries can be serious, taking months to heal.

A bowed tendon is the result of a severe strain of the superficial digital flexor tendon. This tendon is the outermost one at the back of the lower leg, running from the knee down to the pastern. Inflammation from the strain causes pain, heat, and swelling. Fluid leaks into the tissues around the tendon. The amount of tissue damage that occurs depends on the severity of the injury and on how it is treated. As the injury heals, scar tissue replaces normal tendon tissue and interferes with the normal function of the tendon. Repeated episodes of tendon injury result in a permanent bow of the area. The terms *high bow* and *low bow* refer to the area of the tendon affected. Racehorses are most often affected by bowed tendons, but the injury can happen to any horse.

When a tendon injury first occurs, apply cold water or ice packs immediately to prevent inflammation and swelling from becoming severe. Keep the cold on the leg for twenty minutes at a time, and apply a supportive padded wrap between sessions.

Your veterinarian will perform a careful exam that might include ultrasound to view the injury. You'll then receive specific instructions on how long to continue the cold therapy and on the particular type of wrap necessary for your horse's injury. Some type of anti-inflammatory will be administered to your horse. While you notice that this medication reduces pain, your vet uses it to reduce inflammation and prevent further injury to the tendon.

The injured tendon will never be as strong as before it was injured.

The amount and type of use the horse can undergo depends on the severity of the injury. The best way to monitor the tendon's strength is with ultrasound; periodic ultrasound examinations will help you decide how to proceed with your training program without risking reinjury.

A sprain is a stretch or partial tear of a ligament. Ligaments are fibrous bands that connect bones and support the horse's joints. The ligament can be injured when a twisting or pulling force is applied to the joint. Severe sprains can cause a fracture if a small piece of bone is pulled off at the ligament's attachment.

Ligamentous injury can be more severe than a muscle or bone injury because ligaments don't heal very well. They have a poor blood supply and cannot grow to replace themselves once torn. Instead, a scar is left, which is a weak area prone to reinjury.

Two ligaments that are commonly injured are the check ligament and the suspensory ligament. The check ligament is a branch of the deep digital flexor tendon that attaches to the back of the knee. The suspensory ligament runs from behind the horse's knee (just beneath the flexor tendons), down to the fetlock, or ankle joint. There it divides into two branches that cross to the front of the pastern. Stretching or tearing either ligament can lead to severe lameness. You may or may not notice any swelling, but you can sometimes feel enlargement of the ligament with careful palpation. Your horse will show obvious soreness over the area.

Other sprains cause heat, swelling, and pain around a joint. Sometimes there is no way to tell the difference between a severe sprain and a fracture by its outside appearance. Your priority in either case is to prevent the horse from injuring itself further. Apply ice or hose the area with cold water while you wait for the veterinarian. Don't allow your horse to walk on the leg any more than is necessary. Your veterinarian probably will radiograph (X-ray) the area, then apply a strong supportive wrap.

Curb is a thickening of the plantar ligament that runs along the back of the hock. Inflammation of the ligament occurs in horses with poor conformation or after an injury. In severe cases, the bone underneath the ligament becomes inflamed and thickened. During the acute, inflammatory stage of curb, the area should be iced down and wrapped; after healing, the thickening remains, but the horse may not be lame.

Broken Bones

Long gone are the days when a fractured leg spelled immediate doom for the horse. Many small fractures heal nicely, and sometimes even severe breaks can be treated successfully.

A minor fracture may be mistaken for a sprain or strain since the horse can sometimes bear weight on the leg and may not be very lame. Your veterinarian will radiograph suspicious areas to find small fractures.

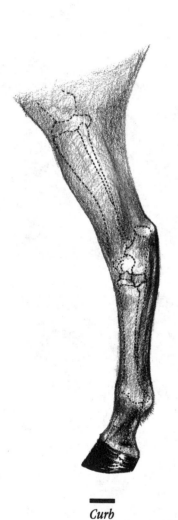

Curb

162

Easy Health Care
For Your Horse

If a fracture is obvious to you, though, it's probably severe. You'll see protruding bone or a funny angle in the horse's leg, or your horse just won't put any weight on the leg. Your first thought should be to prevent further injury to the horse. Do not allow the horse to walk on the leg at all. Wait for the vet to arrive and apply a splint or cast before moving the horse.

You won't be able to do much in these cases, but keeping yourself and the horse calm will be enough. Do not attempt to apply a splint yourself unless you've had special training; an improperly applied or loose splint can be worse than none at all.

Foot Problems

Sudden lameness can also be caused by problems in the horse's feet. After you palpate the leg to eliminate other possibilities, feel the pastern area for increased warmth. Lay the back of your hand on the pastern area. Become aware of the normal amount of warmth that is present. Try to feel the pulse in the arteries running down the back of the pastern. An increase in heat or pulse strength in the front feet is cause for concern. Compare all four feet if you aren't sure. Remember, however, that on a sunny day black feet will absorb heat and feel warmer than white ones.

Many horse owners mistakenly think that their horse has broken its leg when it suffers from a foot abscess. The area is so painful that the horse may not put any weight on the leg. You may see a small spot along the coronary band where the abscess has ruptured onto the surface. See chapter 7 for more about hoof abscesses and for advice on dealing with punctures in the foot.

Laminitis or founder can also cause sudden lameness. The foundered horse won't hold one leg up in obvious distress. Instead, the horse's front feet will be stretched forward to take the weight off his sore toes, and he may refuse to walk. You might feel increased heat in the feet.

If you suspect that your horse has the symptoms of laminitis or founder, you must call your veterinarian immediately. This is the most important first aid that you can give. (See chapter 7 for more information about laminitis.)

Not-So-Sudden Lameness

Countless injuries and maladies can cause a horse to begin to limp. Sometimes the problem comes on gradually, but you don't notice anything until your horse suddenly worsens. If you have not ridden all winter, you may notice lameness during your first ride of the spring. Or

Injuries and
Lameness

you may have been riding lightly, and then asked your horse to work more strenuously.

How to Locate the Source of a Lameness

How can you spot a mild lameness before it becomes severe? If you've been riding continuously, you may notice a slight change in the way your horse moves. Perhaps your horse resists doing a task he has always performed willingly in the past. Don't ignore these subtle signals. While boredom, overwork, or just an off day may be the cause, your horse may very well have a subtle lameness.

Practice watching horses move to learn how to spot lameness. The guidelines given here are just a start, and a lot more is involved in analyzing equine lameness. If you've mastered the basics and want to know more, study the book *Adams' Lameness In Horses* (see appendix).

It is easiest to see lameness when the horse is trotting. Have a friend lead your horse at the trot, being sure to allow slack in the rope. Use a fence or other horizontal structure in the background for reference.

Start by saying "Right, left, right, left," as the right and left front feet hit the ground. Continue your chant as you look at the horse's head. Do the ears stay at the same level as each front foot lands? If not, when does the head lift? With a front-leg lameness, the head rises when the sore leg bears weight. If the head rises slightly every time you say, "right," then the horse is sore on the right front leg. Another way of looking at this is that the head goes down when the good leg bears weight.

Now watch the horse from the side as it trots by you. Notice whether both front legs extend and flex fully with each stride; are right and left stride lengths the same? The horse that is sore in the heel (as with navicular disease or sole bruising) will have a shortened stride. Some types of muscle soreness may not cause a head bob but will prevent the horse from fully extending the leg.

Hind-leg lameness is more difficult to spot. Watch the horse trotting away from you and concentrate on the hips. Again, repeat "Right, left," as each hind foot hits the ground. The hip on the sore side may "hike" (rise up higher than normal) as the horse bears weight on it. Some lamenesses, though, cause the hip to sink below normal as weight is borne on the sore leg.

Next, watch the hind legs from the side as the horse trots past you. Compare the arc of flight of each foot; do both rise equally off the ground? Is either toe dragging? Soreness in the hock or stifle will prevent a horse from fully flexing its hind leg and can result in toe-dragging.

Easy Health Care
For Your Horse

While you watch either the front or hind legs, compare stride lengths of either side. This may be easiest if you look at the hoof prints left in the ground. The sore leg might have a shorter stride. Some lamenesses are easier to spot when the horse is traveling in a circle or up or down a slope. Try lunging your horse in both directions to help you spot a subtle lameness.

Once you've determined which leg is causing the lameness, try to find the part of the leg that is affected. Pick out the foot and examine it carefully. You may find a bruise, or a small stone may be caught between the hoof and shoe. Then carefully palpate the leg to detect heat, swelling, or soreness.

When should you call the vet about a lameness? Although it's helpful to you to be able to locate a lameness, further investigation is needed to answer your basic question: "When can I ride again?" If you want to ride your horse, you should have even a mild lameness examined so you don't risk worsening the injury. Any lameness that lasts more than a few days should be diagnosed, too. A severe lameness should always be examined by the vet.

Your veterinarian may be able to find the problem quickly if an obvious area of pain or swelling can be found. Hoof testers are used to find soreness in the feet. Sometimes more diagnostic work needs to be done. Nerve blocks can help find the source of a mysterious lameness. The veterinarian injects a local anesthetic over a nerve, deadening the feeling to a particular area. If the horse becomes sound, then the problem area has been found. Radiographs or ultrasound may then be recommended to judge the severity of the injury.

Splints

A splint is a soft swelling or a bony enlargement that occurs between the splint bone and cannon bone. The size of a splint can vary from a tiny bump to a large, ugly swelling, and its effects range from an unsightly blemish to a severe lameness.

A new, acute, or "hot," splint is usually accompanied by heat, swelling, and pain; the horse may or may not be lame. An old "cold" splint is a hard bump or blemish that usually does not cause pain.

Splints can have several causes. The syndrome is common in young horses in which the ligamentous attachment of the splint bone to the cannon bone has not yet hardened into bone. Stretching or tearing of the ligament causes new bone to be laid down, and a firm swelling results. Sometimes, too, the splint bone fractures.

Splints in young horses usually occur on the inside of the front legs, since this area bears the most weight. Certain conformation faults predispose horses to developing splints. Horses with "bench knees" (a condition

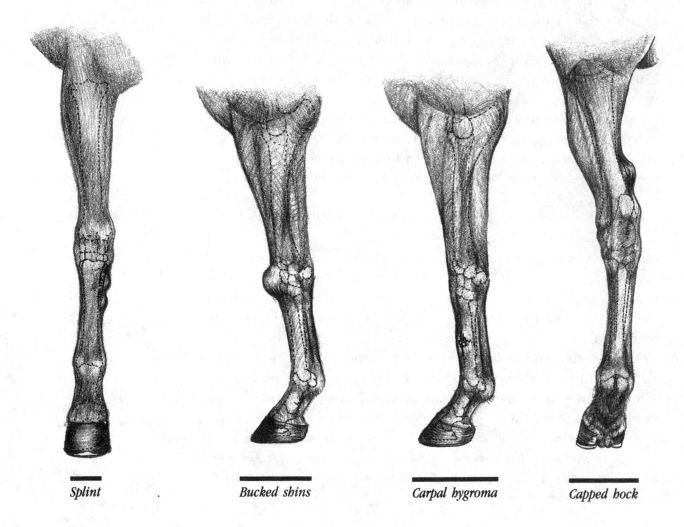

Splint   *Bucked shins*   *Carpal hygroma*   *Capped hock*

in which the knee is offset to the inside relative to the cannon bone) place more stress on the splint bone. The horse with a base-narrow, toed-out stance is prone to hit the inside of one leg with the opposite foot and a cause a splint.

Splints can occur in horses of any age because of trauma or a blow to the leg. Traumatic splints occur on either the outside or inside of the leg, and are just as common on hind legs as on the front.

Always have your veterinarian radiograph (X-ray) the splint to be sure there is no fracture. Some breaks can heal with stall rest, while others require surgery. Young horses can sometimes continue to work if training is gradual and no fracture is found. However, to reduce the size of the lump, allow the horse to rest and wrap the leg until the splint "cools out" (no heat or pain remains). Alternate cold therapy with sweat wraps to minimize tissue reaction and reduce the size of the bump, since the size of the splint can only diminish while the splint is hot. A permanent blemish often remains after the splint has cooled, but the horse is usually not lame.

Easy Health Care
For Your Horse

Large splints can cause lameness even after they are cold if there is enough bone growth to interfere with movement of the ligaments and tendons at the back of the leg. This is less likely to happen if you spot the problem early and take extra precautions to prevent it from progressing.

Bucked Shins

"Bucked shins" is the common term for inflammation of the cannon bone (shin) that occurs in young horses in training. In growing horses, bones strengthen and thicken in response to the stress put on them. If the bone cannot stand up to the stress put on it, microscopic fractures and hemorrhage can occur.

The bucked-shin syndrome ranges from mild soreness to severe lameness with a large, saucer-shaped fracture in the cannon bone. Palpation of the leg reveals heat and soreness at the front of the cannon bone. When this occurs, apply ice, minimize the horse's movement, and call your vet, who will radiograph the leg. Small fractures are difficult to see on an X ray, so several different views must be taken.

Mild soreness is a sign that the horse's bones are not ready for the stress placed on them. Gradual conditioning will prevent a fracture from occurring. Small fractures will heal with stall rest, while larger ones require surgery. Some trainers use various types of heat or counterirritation to try to stimulate faster healing, but it is a matter of controversy whether or not these methods really speed up a return to work.

Soft-Tissue Swellings:
Thoroughpin, Capped Hock, Carpal Hygroma

Soft-tissue swellings can be caused by fluid buildup in a tendon sheath or bursa. A tendon sheath is the thin covering that encases a tendon and normally contains a small amount of lubricating fluid. A bursa is a protective pocket of fluid that forms where a tendon crosses over a bone.

Excess fluid accumulates in these areas because of stress or irritation. Causes include poor conformation, constant trauma (for example, the stall kicker), or an injury. Poor conformation causes extra stress to be placed on the joints, so the horse's body produces excess fluid as a protective measure.

Unfortunately, once an area fills with fluid, it is difficult to get rid of the fluid permanently. (If the cause is poor conformation, the blemish will always be present.) The area tends to fill again even if the fluid is drained. Your chances of eliminating the fluid are better if treatment is

167

Injuries and Lameness

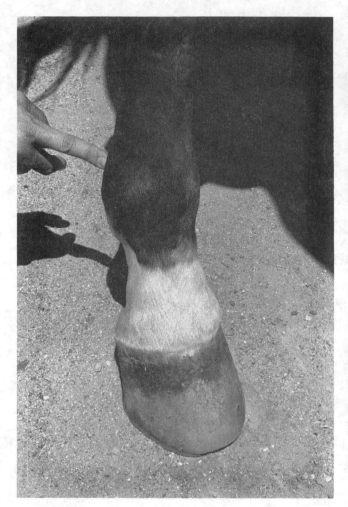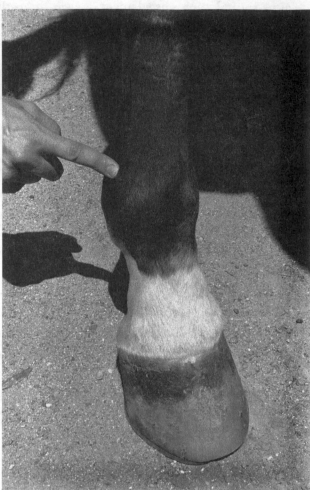

Thoroughpin

Easy Health Care
For Your Horse

sought as soon as you spot the problem. Any of these swellings can be just a bothersome blemish, but your veterinarian may want to radiograph the area to be sure there isn't a bigger problem.

Fluid-filled swellings are named for the areas where they occur. A lump on the front of the knee, caused by fluid in the carpal sheath, is a *carpal hygroma*. A *capped hock* is an inflamed bursa at the point of the hock. With *thoroughpin,* fluid accumulates in the tarsal sheath (the covering of the deep digital flexor tendon); you'll see a swelling behind and above the hock.

A swelling at the ankles because of fluid in the flexor tendon sheath is called *windpuffs*. Articular and nonarticular windpuffs must be differentiated, since nonarticular windpuffs are usually only a blemish. Swelling in the tendon sheath from nonarticular windpuffs occurs between the suspensory ligament and the flexor tendons, just above the sesamoid bones. Articular windpuffs, or swelling in the joint, is discussed below.

You can keep some of these swellings at a minimum by applying sweat or support wraps. Your veterinarian might inject a small amount of a

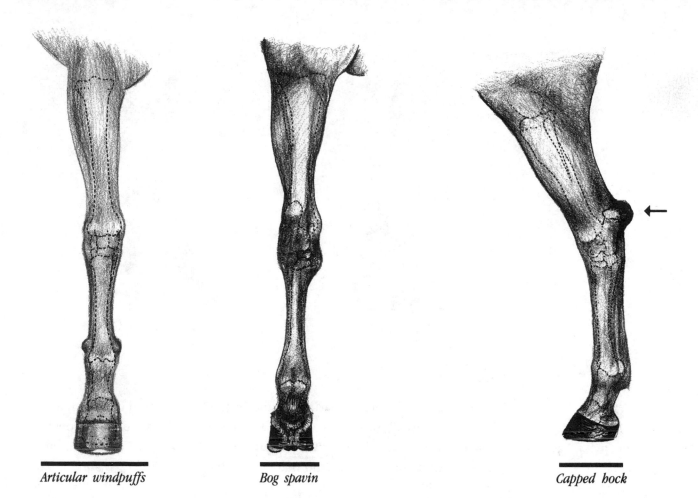

| Articular windpuffs | Bog spavin | Capped hock |

corticosteroid and apply a pressure wrap to prevent the fluid from returning. However, if the cause of the problem is not found, then the condition probably will recur.

Joint Swellings: Articular Windpuffs, Bog Spavin

A swelling around a joint can be only a blemish or it can cause lameness. Your veterinarian will usually recommend that the joint be radiographed to rule out a bone problem; if none is found, you can ride the horse as usual.

Articular windpuffs are swellings of the fetlock joints. In contrast to nonarticular windpuffs, joint swelling is located between the suspensory ligament and the cannon bone, just above the sesamoid bones. Windpuffs usually occur without lameness, but the presence of fluid shows that there is some irritation to the joint. Strenuous training or straight ankles predispose a horse to windpuffs. Once your vet has taken X rays and found no bone abnormality, riding can continue as usual. The amount of fluid can be reduced with pressure or sweat wraps.

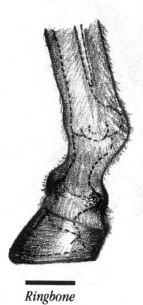
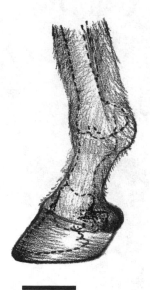

Ringbone   *Side bone*

Bog spavin is an accumulation of fluid in the hock joint. Like windpuffs, bog spavin usually is not accompanied by lameness. However, occasionally a horse will have an underlying defect in the bone. If the horse is not lame and radiographs are normal, then the bog spavin is simply an annoying blemish.

Bog spavin tends to occur in horses with straight hocks, cow hocks (turned in as viewed from the rear), or sickle hocks (in which, when viewed from the side, the rear leg angles forward from the hock down.) Bog spavins in young horses may resolve themselves as the horse grows older. If the blemish is a problem, the fluid can be drained, but recurrence is common.

Arthritis: Ringbone, Sidebone, Bone Spavin

Arthritis usually causes lameness that worsens gradually over a long period. You may not notice the gradual onset, though, but suddenly see that your horse is lame.

Arthritis is a permanent condition, but there are a variety of treatments that can ease the symptoms. Various special shoes, oral medication such as phenylbutazone, or medication injected directly into the joint can help the arthritic horse. Hyaluronic acid and polysulfated glycosaminoglycans (PSGAGs) are used to help slow the progression of arthritis.

Horses can get arthritis in any of their joints, but certain areas are commonly affected and thus have received their own names. High and low ringbone are terms that refer to arthritis in the pastern area. *Low ringbone* is a protruding ring at the coronet that corresponds to arthritis of the coffin joint and short pastern bone. *High ringbone,* which occurs at the pastern joint (between the long and short pastern bones), causes a bulge about an inch above the coronet.

Some cases of ringbone causes severe lameness while others don't seem to bother the horse very much. Radiographs will reveal how much of the bony growth involves the joint, and whether any ligament attachments are involved.

Sidebone is bone growth on either side of the coffin bone. The growth may occur on one or both sides of each front foot. Sidebones don't usually cause lameness.

Bone spavin is arthritis in the hock joint. Certain types of work and conformation predispose the horse to bone spavin. Jumpers, and cutting or roping horses put extra stress on the hock joint. Horses with sickle hocks or cow hocks are also predisposed to bone spavin.

Navicular disease is a degenerative condition affecting the navicular bone within the foot. This disorder, which is not a true arthritis, is discussed in chapter 7.

Osselets is the name used for arthritis of the fetlock (ankle) joint. The ankles of a horse with osselets may look bigger or rounder than usual. *Green osselets* refers to inflammation without bone changes on an X ray. Racehorses are most often affected with osselets because their work places great strain on the ankles.

Exercise-Associated Problems

Heat Exhaustion

Heat exhaustion and heat stroke occur in hot, humid environments when horses exercise heavily. Electrolyte imbalances contribute to the problem. If you work your horse on hot days, make it a habit to check his temperature, pulse, respiration, and capillary refill time after every workout.

You'll find that your horse normally has a slightly increased temperature immediately after exercise. An increased pulse rate and respiratory rate are also normal. The most important guide to your horse's health is the time it takes for these rates to return to their resting values after the workout is finished. The pulse, respiration, and temperature should be near normal within ten minutes of the time you stop exercising.

A typical horse worked on a hot day might finish with a temperature of 102 to 103°F, a pulse rate of eighty to one hundred beats per minute, and a respiration rate of sixty breaths per minute. Panting can be normal since horses cool themselves through air flow in the lungs. Within ten minutes, the horse's temperature should be 101°F, his pulse less than seventy, and his respiratory rate below forty.

A temperature, pulse, or respiratory rate that remains high after ten minutes is cause for concern. Also be concerned if the horses's temperature is over 103°F immediately after exercise. Either your horse was not fit enough for the exercise, or he's overheated, or both.

Hose down your horse's legs with cold water. Keep him in the shade, and put a wet towel on his neck and head. Allow him to drink lukewarm water in small amounts at a time.

Examine your horse's gums. Pink gums with a capillary refill time of two seconds or less (see "The Physical Exam," above), are reassuring. A pale or blue color and a longer refill time should give you cause for concern.

You can prevent heat prostration in your horse by working him in the early morning or late evening on hot days. A gradual training program will allow his body to become used to dealing with the heat, and he will sweat more efficiently.

Be sure your horse has access to a trace-mineral salt block, and ask your veterinarian about the best type of electrolyte supplement for your sport (see "Nutritional Supplements," chapter 2). Give extra electrolytes on hot days and after hard workouts.

After exercise, routinely cool down your horse with a hose bath and slowly walk him until he's dry. Stay in the shade if possible.

Thumps

"Thumps," or *synchronous diaphragmatic flutter* (SDF), is an abnormality that occurs during and after exercise. You'll see a twitching of the horse's flank with each heartbeat. Sometimes the twitching is mild, or it can be severe and accompanied by other signs of heat exhaustion. Loss of electrolytes (such as calcium, sodium, and chloride) in the sweat predisposes the horse to thumps. Low blood calcium is the main culprit.

Normal horses will pull extra needed calcium from their bones after their blood calcium levels drop. Horses with recurrent SDF may have difficulty mobilizing extra calcium from their bones. Ironically, a high-calcium diet (alfalfa hay) is often associated with thumps. Apparently horses that eat a high-calcium diet lose their natural ability to mobilize calcium from their bones. Your veterinarian will help you revise the horse's diet to prevent problems.

A mild case of thumps will go away on its own if you allow the horse to rest. Severe cases are treated with intravenous fluids that contain calcium and other electrolytes. To help you decide whether your horse needs veterinary attention, examine the horse as discussed for heat exhaustion.

Easy Health Care
For Your Horse

Muscle Disorders

"Tying up," "Monday morning disease," *azoturia* or *exertional rhabdomyolysis* are all names for abnormal muscle damage that occurs with exercise. The names describe symptoms of many different diseases with several different causes.

Symptoms of a muscle disorder can be so mild they're hardly noticed, or so severe that hospitalization is needed. Some horses cramp during exercise, becoming stiff, moving with a shortened stride, and perhaps refusing to go on. Other cases occur after exercise. It is easy to confuse the symptoms of tying up with those of mild colic.

Mild sore muscles can occur in any horse; for example, occasional stiffness occurs after a long trail ride or a difficult workout. Simple muscle soreness can be treated with massage, liniments, and rest. If the problem recurs, call your veterinarian.

The severe "tying-up" syndrome most often occurs in heavily muscled mares and fillies, especially Quarter Horses. The syndrome often occurs in horses that receive large amounts of grain. In severe tying up, the horse sweats profusely and its muscles feel hard and warm to the touch. The muscles over the hip are often affected. Breakdown of muscle tissue releases a product called myoglobin; myoglobin causes the urine to turn brown and may result in kidney damage.

A horse that is severely affected must be treated by a veterinarian. Horses with mild but recurring symptoms or horses that do not recover quickly should also be examined. Do not walk your horse during a severe episode, since symptoms could worsen.

Prevention and treatment of tying up start with a specific diagnosis of its cause. Your veterinarian will ask detailed questions about your horse's management to help identify the problem. Among the questions your vet may ask is, are the horse's exercise and feeding schedules consistent? The syndrome called "Monday morning disease" is named after a condition that once commonly affected work horses. After a hard week's work, horses were stabled for the weekend but continued to receive their full ration of grain. When the horses returned to work on Monday morning, some would suffer from muscle cramping.

Feeding the same amount each day, no matter what work the horse does, can contribute to a muscle problem. Horses should be fed and exercised consistently. If the level of exercise changes, so should the amount of feed.

Has the horse had previous episodes of muscle cramping? Some horses, like some people, simply aren't in shape. Perhaps the animal is just not ready for the tasks you present. Even a physically fit horse may have trouble on hot days or at high altitude.

Lack of training must be distinguished from other, more serious muscle disease. Horses that are unfit will not have a history of continual muscle problems. Their soreness and cramping are usually a one-time event that can be prevented by attention to a training program. Be sure you have an adequate warm-up and cool-down period each time you ride, and gradually increase the amount of work your horse does.

Endurance horses (or horses doing any other long-term workouts) occasionally suffer from muscle cramping due to electrolyte loss. Horses lose large amounts of sodium, chloride, potassium, and calcium in their sweat. The risk of illness increases with high temperatures and high humidity.

Does the condition occur at the beginning of exercise? Horses that continually become sore or cramped during exercise might have a defect in the way their muscles work, in the muscle cell membrane, or in electrolyte balance or function within the muscle.

There are several tests that your veterinarian can do to help diagnose the cause of your horse's muscle cramping. Your vet will take blood and urine samples for a complete blood count and a series of biochemical tests. Samples are taken both before and after exercise. A muscle biopsy might be done to help make a specific diagnosis.

Many different remedies have been tried to prevent tying up. Little is known about how, or if, any of these work. Since there are many causes of tying up, you are playing a hit-or-miss game if your horse's specific problem cannot be diagnosed. Your veterinarian may recommend that you stop feeding grain altogether or that you adjust your feeding schedule. You may be told to switch from alfalfa to grass hay.

Electrolyte replacement helps horses that tie up from sweating and electrolyte loss. All horses should have access to a trace-mineral salt block. Endurance rides, competitive trail rides, and field trials are all events where horses are prone to electrolyte losses. If you are involved in one of these sports, ask your veterinarian to recommend an electrolyte supplement or to give you a recipe for an electrolyte mixture that you can administer during competition. (See chapter 2 for details.)

Sodium bicarbonate, or baking soda, is used for some horses. Thiamine or thyroid hormone have eased a few horses' symptoms. MSM (methyl sulfonyl methane) and DMG (dimethyl glycine) are popular but unproven treatments (see chapter 10).

Selenium and vitamin E injections or oral supplements are popular. However, there is little proof showing that low selenium causes tying up, and it is not likely that many causes of tying up in horses will be helped by selenium. In some areas of the country, selenium levels in the feed are higher than needed by the horse (see chapter 2). If you give a selenium supplement in those cases, you could overdose your horse.

Common Emergencies

Eye Injuries and Infections

Eye problems in horses range from simple dust irritation to eyesight-threatening injuries. *Always* call your veterinarian if you suspect a problem with your horse's eyes, since an infection can quickly become severe. Eye injuries or infections are emergencies.

Irritation from dust is a common cause of discharge from horse's eyes. The amount of discharge will increase on hot or windy days, but there will never be a large amount and both eyes will look similar. The horse will not squint and no redness will be apparent. You can safely flush your horse's eyes with sterile saline to remove dust and relieve minor irritation. Don't use a medicated product regularly, since overgrowth of yeasts or fungi can occur.

Simple irritation must be distinguished from an infection, injury, or corneal ulcer. In contrast to the dust-irritated eyes, an infected or injured eye is red, painful, and weepy. An ulcer or scratch on the cornea looks like a white spot on the front of the eyeball.

An *ulcer* is an erosion on the surface of the cornea that results from injury or infection. (See chapter 1 for a review of parts of the eye.) Your veterinarian uses a dye called fluorescein to determine whether the cornea is ulcerated or has been scratched.

Infections or scrapes of the cornea require diligent treatment. Antibiotic ointments or drops last only a few hours after they are placed on the eye, so you must treat your horse frequently throughout the day and night. Your veterinarian telling you to apply a medication every two hours doesn't mean that you can stop at bedtime. Once the problem is under control, treatment intervals may lengthen to every four or six hours.

Deep cuts or severe infections on the eye require surgery. Your veterinarian may take a sample from the infected area for bacterial culture, then sew the eye shut to create a natural bandage. A protective contact lens is temporarily applied in other cases. A small tube can be sewn into the horse's eyelid so that medication is easily applied.

What if you suspect that something is stuck on your horse's eye? If your horse will allow it, rinse the eye out with sterile saline. Small dust particles will wash out easily, but you'll need help to remove larger objects.

Unless your horse is unusually docile, don't risk worsening the problem by trying to grab the object with tweezers; you may accidentally scrape the eye. Your veterinarian will apply a soothing anesthetic to aid in a closer look at the problem.

"Moon blindness" can affect one or both eyes. Also called *periodic ophthalmia* or *recurrent uveitis,* this inflammation of the inner eye tends to recur periodically. Sometimes the cause can be found, but more often it is never discovered. Bacteria, a virus, or a reaction by the horse's body against its own tissues are all possible causes.

Signs of moon blindness include squinting and discharge from one or both eyes. The cornea may change from its normal clear appearance to a milky white, while the conjunctiva become red and irritated.

Moon blindness must be treated every time it occurs. Inflammation inside the eye can cause scarring that interferes with the horse's sight. After checking to be sure that no injury has occurred, your veterinarian will give you two or more medications to apply. A corticosteroid is used to reduce the inflammation and prevent scarring. *Never* use this medication until your veterinarian has first determined that no injury or infection is present, since infection could worsen.

Another medication frequently used for eye infection or inflammation works to dilate the pupil. Scarring could result in the pupil's becoming stuck in one position, and keeping the pupil open helps prevent this scarring and loss of sight. Since the horse will not be able to reduce its pupil size in response to bright sunlight, the animal being treated for eye problems should be kept in a dark stall during the daytime.

Allergic Reactions

Horses, like people, can suffer from allergic reactions. Some allergies occur slowly over time and are not emergencies. These include heaves (an allergic respiratory condition), and itchy skin due to hypersensitivity to the *Culicoides* gnat.

With hives, a suddenly appearing allergic reaction, the horse breaks out in itchy bumps all over its body. Mild cases need no treatment, but call your vet if the horse might injure itself by scratching or if the swelling becomes severe (see chapter 6).

Other allergic reactions occur suddenly and can be life-threatening. Anaphylactic shock is a sudden and severe allergic reaction that occasionally occurs in horses following an injection. The horse collapses, its gums become blue, and its breathing labored. Sometimes the horse rears upward first, or throws itself about.

A similar reaction occurs when an I.V. injection is accidentally given into an artery. The reaction occurring after an intra-arterial injection is immediate, while the anaphylactic reaction occurs about a minute after an injection.

Don't worry about figuring out which problem was the cause of your horse's reaction. The very first thing to do if you see a horse start to react is to *get out of the way*. You can be seriously injured by the horse, and there is absolutely nothing you can do to help. If the horse is in a stall, quickly latch the door to keep him in a confined area and thus reduce his chances of further injury. Your vet will treat the anaphylactic reaction with an injection of epinephrine, antihistamines, or corticosteroids.

Snakebite

Snakebites occur in pastured horses, on trail rides and during camping trips. Bites occur most often on the head, after the horse accidentally grazes near a snake or curiously sniffs at one. A snakebite can be life-threatening. Snakes do not always inject the same amount of venom, so you cannot predict which bites will become serious. Learn about the poisonous snakes in your area so you can easily identify and avoid them.

Snake venom affects the horse in two ways. First, tissues swell and die in the area of the bite. The swelling that you see immediately after the bite proceeds to tissue death and sloughing (the tissue decomposes and falls off) that can take months to heal. Second, venom is absorbed into the bloodstream, where it affects the horse's circulatory system.

The amount of time that passes between a snakebite and veterinary treatment affects the amount of tissue damage that occurs. Your vet will administer anti-inflammatory drugs to reduce swelling, antibiotics to prevent infection, and a tetanus booster. Antivenin might be given if it is available and if the bite has just occurred. Severe bites require intravenous fluids and other treatment for shock.

While you are waiting for the veterinarian to arrive, you can apply cold water packs to the bite to reduce swelling. Keep your horse calm and quiet, since exercise will tire him and can cause increased absorption of the venom into his bloodstream.

If your horse's nostrils appear to be swelling shut, apply the garden hose trick: cut two pieces of hose about six inches long and insert one into each nostril to keep the airways open for breathing.

If you are out on the trail somewhere, use your common sense and judge the situation on its own. If you stay where you are, the horse could become worse; intense exercise (galloping home) could be equally dangerous. If the situation allows, apply cold to the area and proceed slowly toward home.

No matter what new emergency you may face, you'll handle the situation like a pro if you have prepared your first aid kit ahead of time, have practiced applying leg wraps, and are efficient at performing your physical exam. Ask your veterinarian to give a seminar on first aid to you and your friends so you can practice these needed skills.

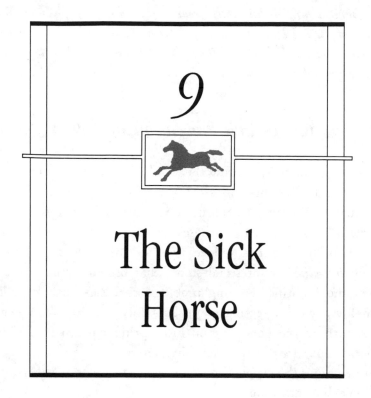

9

The Sick Horse

"A.D.R." is the veterinarian's shorthand for "Ain't Doing Right." Sometimes your horse just isn't quite normal, but you can't figure out what could be wrong. Perhaps your horse has less energy than usual, is losing weight, or didn't eat his evening meal.

Take a closer look to find out the cause. Your horse could have a mild episode of colic or could be coming down with a respiratory virus.

Colic

The bay gelding stretched uncomfortably, a slight twinge in his gut becoming sharper. That morning, the substitute barn man had negligently tossed a moldy flake of hay into the rack. Now he walks by, gives a quick glance, and shrugs. "Must be a little off since the folks are gone," he thinks casually before leaving for the day.

By the time evening feeding rolls around, the gelding is obviously sick. The combination of searing heat and lack of appetite has caused him to become dehydrated, and his bowels have slowed their normal movement. The gelding is rolling on the stall floor when the vet finally arrives.

Causes and Prevention of Colic

What exactly is colic? We throw the word around as if everyone has the same understanding of this "disease." Yet colic is a general term that can apply to many different situations. Colic describes any incident causing pain in the horse's abdomen. Its causes can range from a long-term build-up of sand in the gut to a sudden twist of the intestine. Some horses develop an *enterolith,* or intestinal stone, that becomes stuck in a narrow portion of the intestine. Feeding problems that can cause colic include eating moldy hay or overeating grain. Suddenly switching to a new batch of hay or turning the horse out on lush spring pasture can bring on a colic episode too. In the winter, colic can result from decreased water intake. Impactions (blockages) are more likely to occur at this time, since horses don't like drinking icy cold water. Dry intestinal contents can build up in the horse's large intestine, causing partial or complete blockage.

A twisted intestine can cause severe pain and sudden signs of colic. No one knows exactly how or why twists happen. Many may be related to improper intestinal function that results from parasites or nutritional factors. Horse's bodies were made to process grass taken in by grazing all day; perhaps we upset the intestinal function by feeding separate meals made of hay, grain, or processed feeds.

Parasites can also be a source of colic trouble. Worms can cause permanent but unseen damage, even after deworming. Certain sections of the horse's intestine may never regain normal function. The horse may look just fine, but its intestine isn't clearing out any sand as well as before, and a flake of moldy hay may not be tolerated.

While you can't prevent every incident of colic, you can prevent many of its causes. Start with a good deworming program, giving your horse a product recommended by your veterinarian every two months.

Be consistent in how and what you feed your horse. If you buy a new batch of hay, mix it with the old hay for a few days rather than suddenly switching to the new feed. Keep grain far away from your horse to prevent the slightest chance of accidental overeating.

You can prevent wintertime colic, too. Get a heater for your horse's water supply. There is a variety of models, many of which are inexpensive

Easy Health Care
For Your Horse

and easy to set up. (Be sure to protect any electrical cords from possible chewing by your horse by burying them or running them through a piece of pipe.)

Using a laxative under your veterinarian's supervision can help to prevent colic in a horse that is prone to problems in winter. Any laxative is safest when used intermittently rather than daily. Psyllium fiber (Metamucil) is a good, safe laxative for horses. Bran is another popular laxative that works better when fed once weekly rather than every day. Bran contains high levels of phosphorus and protein, so you don't want to feed very much of it or you'll upset your horse's nutritional balance.

Some horses appear to be predisposed to developing enteroliths (intestinal stones). Preliminary studies suggest that enterolith formation stops when the diet is acidified by adding vinegar. Your vet will tell you if this is necessary.

Signs of Colic

Colic symptoms can range from so mild that they're hardly noticeable to obvious rolling and signs of pain. The earlier you notice your horse's colic episode, the better his chances of recovering without incident.

Early signs of colic are mild and easily overlooked. A horse with mild colic may simply lie down more than usual, or frequently stretch, yawn, and look at his side. Some horses just lose their appetite and mope around, but as pain progresses, the horse paws the ground, kicks at his belly, then begins to roll to try to ease his discomfort.

You may not recognize the early symptoms of colic, or you may mistake those signs for another problem. But you can learn how to evaluate your horse's vital signs so that you can call for help when it's needed. Don't ignore the warning.

The degree of pain a horse shows is not always related to the severity of the colic episode. Simple gas can be extremely painful, while a deadly buildup of sand may cause a gradual onset of dull pain.

The Colic Exam

No matter what you think your horse's problem is, you must be sure to do a thorough exam, or else risk missing an important signal. (See chapter 8 "The Physical Exam".) Begin by taking the temperature, pulse rate, and respiratory rate. Your horse's pulse and respiration will increase in proportion to the amount of pain he's feeling and the extent of internal injury.

Next, look at your horse's mucus membranes. Lift the lip and examine the gums. Are they pink and moist? Check the capillary refill time.

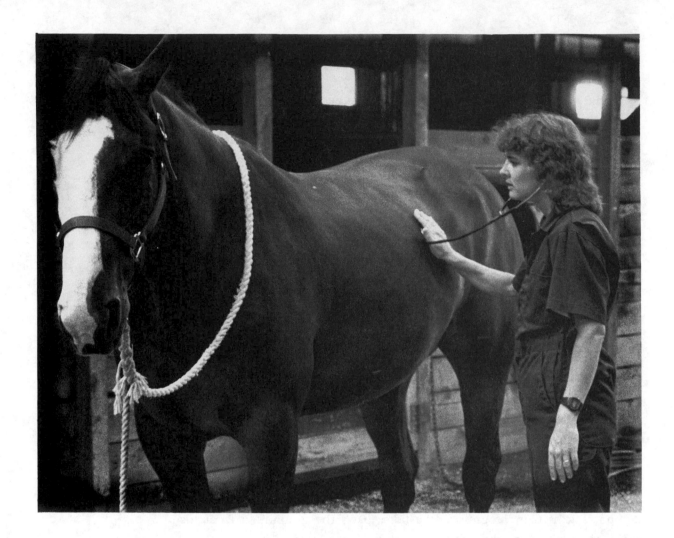

Gums that feel dry, look pale or bluish, or have a prolonged refill time are giving you a clear signal to call the veterinarian immediately.

With your veterinarian's help and lots of practice, you can learn to evaluate your horse's intestinal sounds. Don't expect to figure it out overnight, though. A stethoscope is the best instrument to use, but simply laying your ear against the horse's side can reveal a medley of sounds.

The normal horse's gut has a progressive gurgling sound most of the time. The noise will increase after eating and decrease after exercise. Practice listening to gut sounds at various times of the day so you know the normal variation. Listen on both sides and in various parts of the abdomen. Be sure your surroundings are quiet, or you won't hear a thing.

With colic, the horse's gut sounds may be abnormally silent due to lack of intestinal motility. In other cases there may be loud gurgling because of indigestion caused by overeating lush pasture, suddenly changing feeds, or getting into some moldy hay.

Easy Health Care
For Your Horse

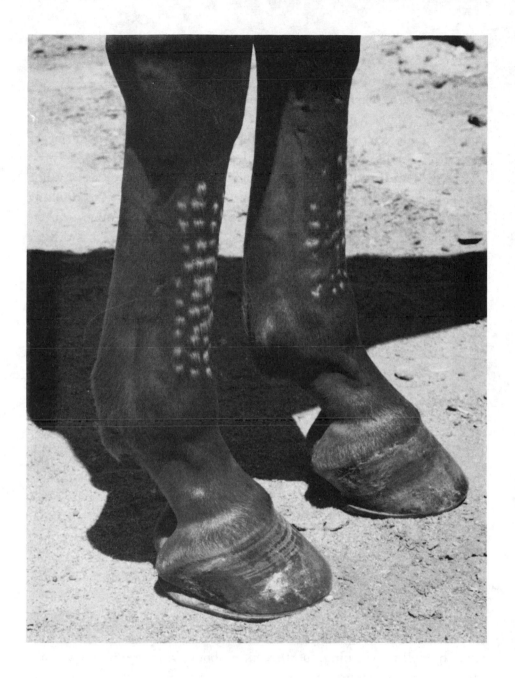

Examining your horse's manure is an important part of the colic exam. You must rely on daily manure cleanup to tell whether today's manure is different from any other. Has your horse passed a normal amount of manure? Is it dryer or softer than normal? Dry manure can signal dehydration or warn of a possible impaction. Soft mature (cow-pie consistency) can occur from indigestion, or it can be normal in horses that eat rich alfalfa hay or graze on lush pasture. Diarrhea (watery manure) in the horse always indicates a problem.

Sand colic is a common problem in some areas of the country. You can do a simple test to see if there is a large amount of sand in your horse's manure. First, fill a bucket with fresh water. Add several manure balls, making sure that they have no sand on their outsides. Stir the mixture, let it settle for a minute, then pour off the liquid. Any sand that the horse has passed will remain at the bottom of the bucket.

While finding lots of sand is significant, its absence does not rule out sand colic. Many horses with sand colic pass very little sand in their manure. Your veterinarian may be able to hear the sand moving in the gut with a stethoscope or see the sand on a radiograph (X ray).

One final area to check in your physical exam is the horse's feet. While they're a long way from the stomach, you should become used to thinking about feet, because laminitis may result from an intestinal upset or over-eating. Check the front feet for increased heat. (See chapters 7 and 8 for more information.)

Thanks to your exam, your vet can decide how soon the horse must be seen, or may give you instructions on how to proceed until help arrives. Also, you can remain calm since you'll have a better idea of what's happening with your horse.

First Aid for Colic

You must call your veterinarian when colic occurs. Even a colic episode that seems mild can progress to severe illness; don't wait until then to call for help. If your horse is not in extreme discomfort, take a few moments to go through your physical exam before making the call. Your vet may give you specific instructions based on what you can relate.

The traditional approach to colic has been to walk the horse—you may have wondered why? Before you automatically begin to walk your horse, remind yourself of what walking will accomplish.

Your horse may be extremely restless with a painful colic episode. To prevent further injury, you'll want to walk a horse that might injure itself by rolling, kicking, or thrashing about. A horse with gas colic might relax enough to pass some of that gas after a long slow walk. Walking probably helps distract the horse's attention from his pain, and the slow walking, with frequent stops, may help the bowels to regain normal activity.

On the other hand, a colicky horse that is standing quietly may become exhausted from extensive walking, or may become overheated on a warm summer day. Exercise also causes a decrease in intestinal motility and sounds. Often the vet arrives to find a sweaty, panting horse, and finds it difficult to decide whether the colic or the vigorous walking has caused those signs. If you're nervous (who wouldn't be?), make sure that you aren't releasing that nervous energy by walking your horse to exhaustion.

What else can you do? Most veterinarians recommend that you remove the horse's hay and grain. While you may be relieved that your horse shows signs of an appetite, taking in more feed could worsen his symptoms. Do, however, allow your horse to drink small amounts of water.

Leave further treatment to the veterinarian. Some horse owners are tempted to administer their own medication before calling for help, reasoning that the vet would give the same drug. Yet while the veterinarian often gives an injection of an anti-inflammatory or painkilling medication, treatment doesn't stop there.

Giving an injectable medication without giving an oral treatment may relieve the horse's symptoms for a time, but the problem won't necessarily go away.

If you have medications on hand, consult your veterinarian before you administer anything. The drug could mask signs of colic, causing your vet to underestimate the severity of the problem. The progression of your horse's symptoms before and after administration of medications is extremely important in evaluating the colic episode.

Treating Colic

After giving the horse a painkiller or antispasmodic, your veterinarian usually gives an oral medication through a stomach tube. Mineral oil, warm water, or a laxative may be administered. In all but the worst cases, these medications help soothe the pain and return the intestinal function to normal.

Surgery is necessary to untangle a twisted intestine or remove a stubborn impaction. Survival rates after colic surgery have improved dramatically in the past several years, but it is still a very expensive operation.

Make your decision about surgery before the question arises so you don't have to do so under pressure. If surgery is necessary, it's usually an emergency. You cannot adopt a wait-and-see approach when your vet recommends an operation, because the horse becomes sicker and the surgery more risky as each minute passes.

Medical treatment of colic is not always cheaper than surgery. Sometimes intensive-care treatment continues for several days. Communication with your veterinarian is essential to make the right decision for you and your horse.

Choke

Signs of Choke

Choke is a common affliction related to the horse's eating habits. The first time you see a choking horse, you probably will get quite a scare. The horse may be frightened too.

Choke occurs when a ball of food sticks in the esophagus, the tube leading to the stomach. Try as it might, the horse cannot get the feed all the way down. Saliva continues to be produced, and the horse drools excessively. You may see green feed coming out of the nostrils.

The horse may panic, throwing itself about and trying to rid itself of the annoyance. Or it may continually stretch out its neck, drooling all the while. Remember, though, the horse can still breathe. The food is lodged in the esophagus, not the windpipe.

Causes, Prevention, and Treatment of Choke

When your horse chokes, your first reaction should be a calm one. Your horse can still breathe since there is no blockage of the airway. Keep your horse calm and prevent him from injuring himself by slowly walking or by standing with him and talking calmly.

Sometimes you can see a lump on the side of the horse's neck where the ball of food is stuck in the esophagus. You may try to massage the throat area to help move the bolus of food down. (The veterinarian will remove the blockage by helping it to pass to the stomach, not by bringing it back up.)

Choke usually occurs because the horse doesn't chew and lubricate his food properly before swallowing, so the food cannot pass normally. A greedy eater is the usual victim of choke. Also, horses that are fed in groups may eat faster than usual due to competition for feed, and so suffer from choke. Horses trying to eat in a swaying trailer can choke when they accidentally swallow a bolus of food before they are ready. Finally, the horse that is overdue to have its teeth floated is a prime candidate for a choke episode; the feed just can't be chewed normally.

Most cases of choke can be prevented. If you feed horses in a group, provide several feeding areas to reduce competition for feed. Avoid feeding grain in a trailer, since grain is more likely to cause choke than is hay (do not provide any feed in the trailer to a horse that gobbles its feed or has a history of choking).

The greedy eater is the horse that is most difficult to protect from choke. Several methods have been tried, and one may work for a particular horse but be useless for another. Feed hay before grain, so the horse is slightly full and less likely to bolt the concentrated feed. Place large rocks in the grain bucket, forcing the horse to pick its way around the rocks to eat the grain. Finally, spread out the feed over a large area to prevent the horse from gulping it down.

Yearly dental exams ensure that the horse's teeth are in good shape and can perform their needed function. Horses with teeth in very poor condition can be given specially prepared feed.

Respiratory Disease

Signs of respiratory disease include nasal discharge (runny nose), coughing, increased breathing rate or difficulty in breathing, fever, and depression. After you complete your routine examination (see chapter 8, "The Physical Exam"), focus on the horse's respiratory system. If you see discharge from your horse's nose, note whether it comes from one or both nostrils. Is the discharge clear, cloudy, bloody, thin, or thick?

If your horse has a cough, when is coughing worse? Does your horse cough during meals, after exercise, at night when you put him into his stall, or all the time?

Is your horse's respiratory rate higher than normal? Watch your horse's flank while he breathes. Is inhaling difficult, or is there a push when he exhales? Are breaths fast and shallow, or slow and deep? As you'll learn from the following sections, the answers to these questions help you and your veterinarian find the cause of your horse's problem.

Infections

A discharge from just one nostril may indicate a sinus infection or a guttural-pouch problem (see chapter 1 for a description of the guttural pouches). Your veterinarian will use an instrument called a fiberoptic endoscope to look into your horse's nasal passages and find the source of the discharge. Both these infections are difficult to treat. Infected guttural pouches must be flushed out each day with an antiseptic solution. Sinus infections usually require surgery to allow drainage.

Bacteria and viruses can attack your horse's respiratory system. Respiratory viruses are common in young horses (see chapter 4). During early stages of illness, your horse may simply look depressed or refuse to eat. Take your horse's temperature and look for signs of nasal discharge from both nostrils or an increased respiratory rate.

Most veterinarians will not prescribe antibiotics for the horse with a mild respiratory virus; the disease must simply run its course. If the horse shows signs of a bacterial infection, though, medication will be given. A high fever, thick nasal discharge, or involvement of the lungs might prompt treatment.

Pneumonia is an infection of the lungs that can be caused by a virus or bacteria. Pleuritis is an infection of the pleura, the lining around the lungs, while pleuropneumonia is inflammation of both the pleura and the lungs. Pneumonia and pleuritis, serious diseases that require several weeks of treatment, can permanently weaken your horse. Severe cases can be prevented by understanding how and why they occur.

There are many causes of pneumonia and pleuritis. Sometimes a viral

The Sick
Horse

infection weakens the lungs and allows invasion by bacteria. Shipping the horse over a long distance can cause enough stress to worsen a normally mild viral infection. A flake of hay is tossed in the trailer, vents are opened for air, and the driver takes off, not realizing that the horse has been set up to get sick. Road dust, exhaust fumes, and mold spores from the hay are all forced into the horse's airway because the vent is opened in front of his face. Since the horse's head is tied, normal flow of mucus up and out of the airways can't occur.

You can prevent problems by keeping vaccinations up to date and avoiding shipping if your horse is even mildly sick. When you do trailer your horse, don't open a vent that will blow air directly into his face. Lack of ventilation is just as bad, however, since humidity inside the trailer increases the number of bacteria in the air. Open vents or windows at the back of the trailer provide good ventilation. Let your horse out after several hours and allow him to graze or offer hay on the ground so that he lowers his head and the airways can drain.

Heaves

"Heaves," "broken wind," or *chronic obstructive pulmonary disease* (COPD) is an allergic type of respiratory disease. Veterinarians compare COPD to asthma, emphysema, or an allergy, because heaves, like human asthma, causes the horse's lungs to become hyperreactive to dust, molds, fungi, or pollens in the air.

The incidence of COPD increases as horses age. Heredity, chronic bronchitis (an inflammation of the airways), or a respiratory virus are possible causes of heaves.

Signs of heaves include a cough, lack of energy, or weight loss. The onset can be so slow that you don't notice your horse's symptoms. Perhaps your horse has been fine all summer, but develops a cough during the winter. You might attribute a horse's lack of energy to age or laziness. Heaves is one cause of poor performance in the athletic horse. You'll see a gradual decrease in energy or athletic ability, or the horse may quickly become short of breath during exercise.

An early sign of heaves is a chronic cough. Some horses cough just after feeding because the dust and molds in hay irritate their lungs. Others cough more often in wintertime because they are enclosed in a stuffy stall. Horses that are worse in the summer are sensitive to dust or pollen in the air.

Sometimes the first sign of heaves is a respiratory infection or pneumonia, since the lungs can't ward off disease normally. Although the infection clears up with antibiotic treatment, the lungs are not normal and the horse is still susceptible to disease.

Horses affected with heaves suffer from spasms of the airways that make

Easy Health Care
For Your Horse

breathing very difficult. Weight loss occurs because the horse must use more energy to breathe. By the time you notice your horse's weight loss and breathing difficulty, the condition has been there for some time.

Airway spasm occurs with expiration, so your horse will inhale normally but exhale with a push. The muscles just behind the last ribs help push air out. These muscles enlarge in what is called a "heave line" after years of use.

Spotting severe cases of heaves is easy, but milder cases are more difficult to diagnose. Your veterinarian will listen to the horse's lung sounds before and after exercise. A fiberoptic endoscope might be used to look into the horse's airways. Mucus samples are taken for laboratory analysis of cell types and numbers, and are cultured to detect the presence of bacteria.

For a more specific diagnosis, your veterinarian runs a series of allergy tests on your horse. The tests are similar to those done in people. The veterinarian injects a small amount of each allergen (allergy-causing substance) under the skin. Injections that cause a reaction are assumed to contain substances to which the horse is allergic, but false positives can occasionally occur. Ask your vet to refer you to someone who is experienced at running the test, if necessary.

Treatment of Heaves

Treatment of heaves is easy to discuss, but much harder to do. Since there is no permanent cure, the best solution is to remove the horse from the environment that causes his symptoms. After allergy testing, specific allergy-causing substances can be removed from the horse's environment. Some horses are especially sensitive to hay; others are allergic to particular grains.

If allergy testing is not done or yields inconclusive results, then you must prevent contact with any dust, fungi, and molds that might trigger your horse's reaction. You can try to experiment to find out what can be causing the problem, but you will be most successful if you assume that everything mentioned above is irritating to your horse. After you make the necessary changes, allow several weeks for your horse's symptoms to subside.

Most horses with heaves have fewer symptoms when turned out to pasture. Paddocks or stalls are dusty, and a closed area contains more mold and irritants than open spaces. Barns with poor ventilation or infrequent cleaning may have high levels of ammonia in the air.

If the horse must stay in a barn, do not use straw for bedding; newspaper or peat moss bedding might be less irritating than straw or shavings. No matter what type of bedding you use, however, thoroughly clean the stall every day. Maintain nearby stalls the same way. The barn must have

The Sick
Horse

a good ventilation system. Hose down open areas of dirt, including paddocks and the arena, to reduce dust.

Keep the horse in a stall or paddock that is as far as possible from the indoor ring or arena. Storage areas for bedding, hay, and straw also should be far from the horse's stall; the affected horse should be kept at least fifty yards upwind of any hay storage area.

Feeding pellets or cubes is better than feeding hay. Wetting down the hay helps in only a few cases, since even the best hay contains millions of fungal spores. If the horse is too thin but is allergic to grain, feed vegetable oil, adding it gradually to allow the horse to become accustomed to the change.

Medical treatment for heaves is sometimes necessary. Corticosteroids are effective, but carry a risk of side effects. Allergy shots can help some horses. Other medications includes bronchodilators, expectorants, mucolytic medications (to loosen sticky mucus), and antihistamines.

If the horse has an infection, antibiotics are prescribed. Anti-inflammatories such as phenylbutazone ease discomfort in certain cases. Some horses improve with frequent vaccination against influenza and rhinopneumonitis. Several different immune modulators have been tried, but none have been proven completely successful.

Your veterinarian will begin treatment based on the severity of your horse's signs and the results of diagnostic testing. You may try several different combinations of medications before you find an effective regimen. Once again, since the problem is not curable, the best solution is to change the horse's surroundings, removing the cause of its symptoms.

Laboratory Tests for Horses

"I don't want to spend any more money than is necessary," my client grumbled. "Why should I have a blood test done on my horse? It's obvious that he just has a cold."

Why, indeed? Many horses suffer brief bouts of the flu or mild cases of colic, recovering quickly without further incident. Your vet comes out, gives some type of medication, and that is all there is to the matter. Or is it?

What about a case of the flu that turns into pneumonia? Or a colic that recurs frequently and mysteriously? At what point should a veterinarian look beyond the physical exam and suggest further testing?

When Is Testing Needed?

The most obvious time for tests is when your horse is suffering from a severe illness. Another time for testing is when a medical problem lasts longer than expected or recurs. Examples include the horse that colics frequently, has recurrent muscle soreness after only light exercise, or loses weight for no apparent reason.

When and how often tests are done also depends on you. Are you comfortable with your veterinarian's "almost sure" diagnosis or would you prefer documented proof? Would you rather use the medication that usually works on most horses with a respiratory infection, or do you want to know what medicine will definitely work?

The results of a test may confirm that you're using the proper treatment. If your horse is the exception to the rule, though, you'll be ahead in time and money because you'll know that the routine medication wouldn't have worked. Perhaps you'll now know to use a different drug, or to give medications over a longer time than was originally planned.

Test results can sometimes leave you frustrated. The results may only confirm your veterinarian's suspicions, leaving you wondering whether the test was really necessary at all. The test results may also all be normal, yet your horse may still have a problem.

In neither of these cases are tests a waste of time. Normal tests results help rule out many different diseases, so your vet can isolate the problem. Moreover, many times both you and your veterinarian need the reassurance that your treatment regimen is correct.

The next time your veterinarian suggests running some laboratory tests on your horse, give considerable thought to the matter. What will the tests do to help your horse? Is further information needed to treat the illness properly? Is your horse's illness severe enough that you need more information quickly? Or is the problem a mild one that gives you the flexibility to wait, deciding on tests only if your present treatment doesn't work? Only by weighing all the factors can you and your vet reach a correct decision.

The CBC

The CBC, or complete blood count, is a test in which the horse's blood cells are evaluated and counted. An increased total white blood cell count may result from stress, inflammation, or infection. A decreased count may mean that the cells are pooling somewhere in the horse's body.

The red blood-cell volume is measured in relation to the horse's plasma volume. The relationship between these is called the hematocrit or packed cell volume (PCV). A high PCV occurs with dehydration or shock; if the PCV is low, the horse may be anemic.

The Sick
Horse

Plasma protein levels are measured next. Protein levels may be high due to chronic inflammation, or low because of diarrhea or other loss.

For the differential white blood-cell count, a drop of blood is smeared onto a slide and stained. The different types of white blood cells are closely examined, and their numbers compared to normal counts. Among these cells are neutrophils, the "pus cells" that come to the rescue when your horse suffers from a bacterial infection; and lymphocytes, whose numbers increase when a virus invades your horse's body. The eosinophil is a brightly staining white blood cell that increases in number in response to allergy irritation, or parasite infestation (worms). Monocytes are formed in higher numbers when a disease has been present for a longer time.

With regard to a respiratory disease, your veterinarian might search for several answers: Is the horse suffering from heaves, an allergic problem? Or does it have a virus, such as influenza? Has the problem existed for some time, gradually creeping up on the horse so you have only recently noticed? Or is it an acute (sudden) illness?

Comparing blood counts several days apart can help your vet evaluate how well your horse is combating the disease and how well the medication is working. For example, a high white blood-cell count from pneumonia should begin to drop after your horse receives antibiotics. If the medication isn't working, the white cell count remains high.

The horse with colic also benefits from the CBC. Test results help the veterinarian to determine how severe the illness is and to select the best treatment. Severe cases of colic will show a high PCV, due to dehydration or shock, and sometimes will have a very low total WBC count. The reason is that the white blood cells are pooling in an injured area of the horse's instestine. A high eosinophil count could show that the cause of the colic episode was intestinal parasites.

Serum Chemistries

Your veterinarian may order a set of serum chemistries from the lab. Your horse's serum, obtained after removing the clot from the blood sample, contains many enzymes, proteins, and other substances. Each of these substances is produced by specific body tissues in particular levels. An increase or decrease in any of the products measured can suggest a problem with a particular part of your horse's body.

For example, a horse suffering from muscle soreness might have an increase in the enzyme creatine kinase (CK) that is produced by normal muscle cells. Bruising or muscle damage from "tying up" can cause an increase in blood levels of CK. As treatment and a specific training schedule are begun, the horse's CK levels are monitored to evaluate how well he is responding.

Many veterinarians recommend a routine chemistry screen for older horses. Some old horses lose weight gradually, and although they might

Easy Health Care
For Your Horse

need dental work or more groceries, there is often more involved. As the horse ages, his kidney and liver function may start to deteriorate. The chemistry screen will reflect those problems, and your veterinarian can make specific recommendations about changes in your horse's diet and management.

Serology

Serology is the study of serum to identify antibodies, which are specific proteins produced by the horse's body to help fight disease. Sometimes serology is the only way to diagnose a horse's illness.

Potomac horse fever, influenza, rhinopneumonitis, and equine infectious anemia (EIA) are diseases commonly diagnosed through serology. The test for EIA is familiar to most horse owners as the Coggin's test.

Finding antibodies against a specific disease in the horse's blood is not enough for a diagnosis, since antibodies may be present for a long time prior to the test. Two samples are usually taken several weeks apart, and a sharp rise in the antibody level shows that the infection was very recent.

Other Laboratory Tests

Other fluid and tissue samples can be taken for a detailed look at specific cells, either from a tumor or from body cavities. Horses normally have a small amount of fluid in their chest and abdominal cavities, and a sample can easily be taken.

Fluid is drawn from the horse's abdomen during abdominocentesis. This "belly tap" helps evaluate cases of colic. Thoracocentesis obtains chest (thoracic) fluid for evaluation of respiratory disease. A sample of joint fluid is taken to check for infection or signs of other joint disease. A transtracheal wash obtains fluid and cells from the horse's larger airways, while bronchoalveolar lavage collects samples from deeper in the lungs; both tests aid in the diagnosis of respiratory disease.

The processes used for taking these varied samples are all similar. Skin over the area to be evaluated is clipped and surgically scrubbed before a local anesthetic is injected. Next, a needle, biopsy instrument, or catheter is inserted, and fluid or cells are removed. The amount needed is not large, since a small drop can be placed on a microscope slide and viewed under high magnification.

Your veterinarian usually looks at tracheal washes or abdominal fluid immediately. First, the type and number of cells are examined. A possible finding might be an increase in neutrophils on a tracheal wash, which indicates a bacterial infection. Cells are not the only substances evaluated in these samples; levels of protein, glucose (sugar), and other products are measured as well.

Cultures are sometimes submitted to a laboratory for evaluation of microbial growth. When the type of bacteria causing an infection is known, then the most effective treatment can be chosen. With a culture and sensitivity test, bacteria are grown in the presence of various antibiotics to find the medication that best inhibits that growth.

Other samples are sent to a veterinary pathologist for evaluation. That lump on your horse's skin must be carefully identified so the proper treatment can be given.

Your horse's urine and manure can provide clues to its health, too. Manure is most often evaluated for numbers and types of parasite eggs (see chapter 3). The presence of large amounts of sand in the manure can give a clue to the cause of recurrent colic.

Urine is sent to the lab for bacterial culture if a urinary tract infection is suspected. Urine concentration, or specific gravity, is measured to evaluate kidney function. Cells present in the horse's urine can be examined for evidence of disease.

Although the mainstay of diagnosis continues to be a thorough, accurate physical exam, we can learn much more about the horse's body through a wide array of laboratory and blood tests. The exam determines which, if any, of these tests might help the veterinarian select a better treatment or might help narrow down a specific diagnosis of the problem.

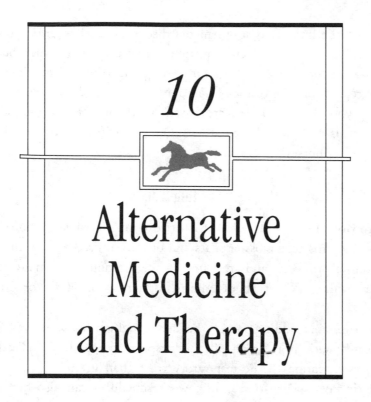

10

Alternative Medicine and Therapy

*Those who fall in love with practice
without science are like a sailor who
enters a ship without a helm or
compass and who never can be certain
whither he is going.*

—*Leonardo da Vinci*

The quest for faster racehorses, better-quality show horses, and more rapid growth of youngsters has led to intense research in equine nutrition, sports medicine, and therapy. At the same time, the public's need for quick cures and better chances at winning has resulted in a large number of dubious products and feed supplements that mainly result in lining someone's pocket.

Remember two things about alternative medicine. First, don't laugh—many of these modalities work. Second, be cynical—alternative medicine can be expensive and is often misused. Reading this chapter will help you determine which products are useful and which are a waste of your time and money.

New Vitamins, Minerals, and Feed Supplements

Are There "New" Dietary Essentials?

Aside from the basic feed supplements discussed in chapter 2, you'll read every so often about a "new" nutrient, "natural" feeds that help your horse's health, or new guidelines for feeding the same old nutrients. Some of these reports are the result of genuine research, and concern topics that can help your horse. Others are based on theory or testimonials ("My horse ate this and won the Kentucky Derby") while no real studies have been done on horses.

Feeding Fat

You probably know that adding a little corn oil to your horse's grain helps to keep his coat glossier. Fats and oils are ingredients in many coat-conditioning products, and are found in small amounts in many commercial grain mixes. What about adding higher levels of fat or oil to the diet?

It appears that adding fat to the diet can help some horses. Fat can help horses with heaves, an allergic respiratory condition. Feeding fat causes less irritation to the respiratory tract than grain.

Athletic horses with demanding work schedules can also benefit from fat if they have trouble taking in enough calories to meet their needs. The horse easily adjusts when the level of fat is gradually increased in the diet, and the danger of colic and founder is much less than if you were to feed the same amount of calories as grain. Fat can be fed at a level as high as 8 percent of the grain mix, or up to one pound daily, if it is introduced gradually into the diet.

What kind of fat should be used? Horses can use both animal and vegetable fats effectively, although corn oil is easier to add to grain than is solid animal fat. Freshness is essential because improper storage of fats can lead to rancidity.

Commercial fat products are available, but choose one with caution. Manufacturers may use special processing so the fat is in a more convenient form, but the effects of this processing on the fat itself are often known to be detrimental or have not been studied. For example, fat is much less digestible when mixed with calcium salts.

Only when all the horse's basic needs are met should feeding fat be considered; it will not compensate for a poor diet or inadequate training.

Laxatives

Laxatives are another type of feed supplement. Bran acts as a laxative by carrying extra water through the digestive tract. Bran contains high levels of phosphorus and protein, and is partially digested by the horse (in contrast to humans, who cannot digest it). You might throw your horse's nutritional balance off by feeding bran continuously or in large amounts. Bran works best as a laxative if it is used intermittently, such as in a once-weekly mash.

Psyllium is used as a laxative to help prevent sand colic. You can use a product intended for humans such as Metamucil, or one of several brands labeled for horses. Your veterinarian will prescribe the amount of psyllium your horse needs and how often it should be given. Horses that have problems with sand colic may need weekly treatments.

Probiotics and Digestive Aids

Several products are marketed as feed additives that will help your horse's digestive system. They are useful for horses that are sick or stressed, but probably won't benefit a healthy horse.

Probiotics are products containing live bacteria. These are marketed with the claim that they aid the horse's digestive system by normalizing the balance of intestinal organisms. Probiotics are most useful for sick horses recovering from colic or diarrhea.

Enzymes are marketed as a digestive aid for horses. These products supposedly help the horse digest his feed more efficiently. Normal horses make their own digestive enzymes in large amounts in the gut, so these products won't add anything new.

Yeast culture and brewer's yeast are two different supplements. Yeast culture is a product containing dried live yeast (single-cell organisms) and fermented grains. Yeast culture is used to increase digestibility and feed efficiency, so it might be helpful for older horses. Also, studies have shown that feeding yeast culture improves the growth rates of foals.

Brewer's yeast consists of dead organisms and is used as a protein and vitamin source. Brewer's yeast is much higher in protein and B vitamins than is yeast culture. However, it does not provide the benefit of increasing feed digestibility.

Natural Foods and Drugs

In today's world of cancer and chemicals, pollution and hazardous waste, everyone wants to live a little more naturally. Many people believe that "natural" products cannot hurt a horse, and that "natural" products are healthier to use than artificial ones. But you might ask, What exactly is "natural"?

There are no laws that govern the use of the word "natural" in equine feeds and supplements, so be careful of commercial products that might take advantage of your desires but do not deliver the result you are after. Some "natural" products contain no additives or preservatives. Manufacturers of other "natural" medications claim their product is obtained directly from nature or is still in plant form. The fine line between "natural" and "synthetic" often cannot be discerned.

Many drugs began as "natural" products, and then were made safer and better by removing the extra parts of the substance that were useless or harmful. Other plants contain drugs or druglike substances in such small amounts that the plant itself is not useful, but a more concentrated "synthetic" product can be made.

Makers of some "natural" products would like you to believe that their supplement is better because it has not been purified, or it contains "unknown micronutrients" that your horse needs. On the contrary, using those unknown nutrients could backfire. For example, high levels of iodine in some products containing seaweed (kelp) caused goiter in horses in the past.

Before you reach for that "natural" product, ask yourself what it is that makes it natural and why it is therefore better. Then find out what the "natural" ingredients are and whether those substances have any pharmacological (druglike) action.

Many "natural" medications, including herbal remedies, are useful, yet they should be recognized for what they are—another type of medication. Plants can contain many substances, ranging from deadly poisons to useful and powerful drugs. These can be overdosed or can cause side effects just as any manufactured drug can. Giving your horse something in plant, herbal, or "natural" form should not lull you into thinking that it is safer than a "synthetic" substance.

What about "natural" feed additives that claim to calm down or perk up your horse? The calming formulas usually contain amino acids and vitamins that are involved in the body's own calming mechanisms. Stimulant formulas contain sugar and vitamins that give your horse a quick burst of energy. These products probably aren't harmful, but it's debatable whether or not they work.

What about immunity-boosting feed supplements? Any horse that is lacking in a particular nutrient will become healthier when that nutrient is given. However, healthy horses won't have greater resistance to disease if they receive more than the recommended daily allowance of nutrients.

Before you buy a "natural" vitamin supplement, decide whether you can achieve the same result by purchasing better-quality feed that contains natural vitamins. For example, green alfalfa hay provides beta carotene, a natural source of vitamin A.

If you really want to stay natural, focus on getting the best-quality hay and grain that you can find, as well as providing the best health care possible. Your horse will be naturally healthy without needing anything else.

A Drug by Another Name:
When Is a Food a Drug?

What about yucca, mussel extract, bee pollen, carnitine, and seaweed? What about "nutrients" you haven't heard of before? Unfortunately, many "nutritional" products for horses are designed for therapeutic uses, but are marketed as supplements. Some of these ingredients are substances used in the horse's body. Any dietary need is unknown since a deficiency for these items has never been determined.

Why do these substances, many of which have been known for years, still carry a "supplement" label? The privilege of using a drug label and making therapeutic claims requires a solid background of research that documents those claims. In addition, FDA approval requires toxicology tests that prove the drug is not harmful at recommended doses. These long, expensive tests are used by manufacturers as an excuse for the lack of FDA approval.

As long as people continue to buy products that haven't been tested, companies won't bother to do research. Companies can market the product as a nutritional supplement, though, and use testimonials (quotes from satisfied users) to describe how the product cures disease or provides some nebulous performance improvement. Look for the difference between testimonials and manufacturers' claims backed by research.

Examples of these kinds of products include DMG (dimethylglycine), marketed as a "health enhancer." Another is MSM (methyl sulfonyl methane), marketed as a sulfur-containing feed additive.

DMG, dimethylglycine, dimethylglyoxine, pangamic acid, calcium pangamate, or vitamin B_{15} are not all the same, although they are related. DMG is promoted as an immunity-boosting substance, but so far there is little evidence showing that it stimulates horses' immunity. DMG and its relatives are marketed as feed additives for horses. However, the FDA does not recognize DMG as a vitamin. More research needs to be done to define how, when, and why it works, its specific effects on horses, and its appropriate dose. In addition, the multitude of products that are called "DMG" must be carefully distinguished, since they are not all the same.

Another chemical in the experimental realm is MSM, or methyl sulfonyl methane. This product is a derivative of DMSO (dimethyl sulfoxide), the malodorous anti-inflammatory (see chapter 4). Proponents of MSM hope that it will provide the same effects as DMSO but without the odor and with an easier, oral route of administration. MSM is marketed as a "sulfur-containing nutritional supplement." Product labels discuss the role that sulfur plays in metabolism. Yet a need for extra sulfur in the horse's diet is questionable. Sulfur in the diet is obtained through proteins, so the horse receiving an adequate level of protein probably takes in enough sulfur.

New Drugs

Jugs, Blood Buildups,
and Bleeding Remedies

"Jugging" a horse means giving a mixture of substances through the jugular vein in the hopes of improving performance. The contents of a jug usually include something colorful, amino acids, vitamins, glucose (sugar), and perhaps electrolytes or minerals.

Horses are given a jug just before a race or show to try to improve their performance. Whether the jug makes any difference is controversial; testimonials abound but proof is scarce.

Blood buildups, or hematinics, are also touted as a boost to the horse's performance. These products, which can be injected or given orally, contain iron, copper, B vitamins, and other elements needed for red blood-cell production. Even though they're widely used, it's controversial whether blood buildups work to increase blood volume, and whether an increase in the red cell volume makes any difference to a horse's performance.

Some racehorses bleed from the lungs during or after racing. "Bleeding remedies" with a supplement label are given to racehorses in the hope that the incidence of bleeding will be reduced. They contain nutrients such as vitamins B complex, C, and K, hesperidins, bioflavonoids, iron, and cobalt. Although the C and B vitamins are probably harmless, other ingredients, including iron, are already in your horse's ration, and you could harm the horse with oversupplementing them.

Whether any of the ingredients in bleeding remedies have anything to do with a horse's bleeding problem is unknown. Many of the ingredients are included because they have been used in humans with bleeding problems. While the cause of bleeding in horses has not been found, it's known that horses do not suffer from many of the bleeding disorders that afflict people, so horses will not necessarily respond to treatments that work on humans.

Immune Modulators

Immune therapy is the use of a substance to help treat, prevent, or decrease the symptoms of disease by affecting the body's immune system. Immune modulators are substances that modulate the immune system, either by stimulating or by depressing the immune response. Some drugs are FDA-approved for use in horses as immune modulators, while others are available as feed supplements.

Immune stimulation can be done in a variety of ways, since the immune system is extremely complex. Your horse's overall health influences how effective his immune system is in accomplishing its task. If your horse has a parasite problem, isn't getting good nutrition, or is under stress, then his immune defenses don't work optimally.

Immune stimulants can be as simple as a nutritional supplement or they can be much more complex, influencing the way your horse's white blood cells work. In a broad sense, vaccinations are a form of immune therapy, since they cause the horse to produce its own antibodies to disease.

An immune stimulant might be used when conventional treatment isn't working as well as expected, if the horse has an ongoing problem that won't clear up, or if you need the horse to return to competition and want to speed up the recovery process. Immune stimulants may also be used to aid recovery from viral infections, since antibiotics are not effective against these organisms. Immune modulators are used in cancer therapy, too.

Vaccinating your horse stimulates its system to make antibodies to that particular disease. However, sometimes antibodies are needed on short notice and a vaccine won't do the job quickly enough. Antibodies can be given to horses in the form of plasma. Plasma donor horses are vaccinated frequently so their blood contains large amounts of antibodies to specific diseases. This concept can be carried further by hyperimmunizing a donor against one specific disease. This hyperimmune serum can then be used for treatment of a horse or foal with that disease.

Interferon is a naturally occurring protein made for medical use by genetic engineering. Each species makes its own specific interferon proteins that work against cancer and viruses. While it is effective, use of interferon is limited by availability and cost.

One group of immune stimulants that has been used for decades are made of bacteria. Injection of these products stimulates the horse's immune system to action. EqStim, BCG, and Ribigen are among the bacterial products used on horses.

EqStim has been used to help treat respiratory disease in horses. Injections must be given intravenously by a veterinarian.

BCG is a vaccine that has been used to treat equine sarcoids (see chapter 6). Ribigen, a more refined product, is also used to treat sarcoids. Injection of an immune stimulant into the area around a sarcoid makes the horse's body react against the growth, so the growth's appearance after injection often becomes worse and then gradually improves.

The way that some substances work isn't completely known. Levamisole, for example, is a deworming medication that seems to stimulate the immune system. In horses, levamisole is sometimes used to help ease the symptoms of chronic respiratory disease (heaves), but inconsistent results have hindered its use.

Immune modulators are used in treating at least one type of equine cancer. The melanoma, a dark-colored growth that occurs most often on

Alternative
Medicine
and Therapy

gray horses, is frequently found around the anal area. Use of a drug called cimetidine appears to assist the horse's natural immune system in destroying the melanoma.

Allergic horses can be treated with immune therapy. Hyposensitization is the use of allergy-causing substances (allergens) to help reduce an allergic reaction. Horses affected with heaves or insect allergies might undergo this treatment (see chapters 6 and 9).

While you need to beware of unfounded claims, the concept of immune therapy is a valid one that will be a part of the future of veterinary medicine.

An Approach to New Ingredients

Rather than list all the new and novel substances you may encounter, let's develop a common sense approach to dealing with the situation.

Many true benefits have been derived from products such as yeast and probiotics. On the other hand, don't assume that all products have undergone rigorous testing. Get the manufacturer's literature to help you evaluate the claims.

Try to recognize your own patterns of thinking that could lead to trouble. Check to see which of the following statements you believe.

If a product has been used on people, it is safe and has been thoroughly tested.

If people widely use a product to achieve a particular effect, that effect has been proven to occur.

If this product has a certain type of effect on people (or another animal), that same effect will be seen in my horse.

There are three possible outcomes of such thinking: a benefit to your horse; a negative effect on your horse; or no effect at all. You can choose to believe that a product works until scientific studies prove that it doesn't. Or, take the opposite stand and assume it doesn't work or is dangerous until you see the studies showing otherwise.

How do new ingredients get into our equine supplements? Many products are used to produce certain responses in people, and so are used in the hope that the same result will occur in the horse. For some products widely used by people, no studies have been done showing that the products work. Popular use is based on rumors and hopes of a particular outcome.

Many products sold as health foods or "natural" therapy for people and later for horses haven't been tested on either animals or people to verify the claims made. Anyone can use the word "natural" on an equine product, since there are no laws concerning that claim. (Only recently has there been a law on the use of the world "natural" for human food.)

Some products have been tested on other animals or on people, and the results are assumed to be the same for horses. There are many cases where this practice is extremely dangerous. One example is monensin, a growth promoter safe for cattle but deadly to horses.

For those ingredients whose affect on the horse is still untested, here are some pertinent questions to ask:

How was the dose for a horse figured? Drug doses are often calculated by weight; a thousand-pound horse receives ten times the dose given to a hundred-pound person. Sounds logical, but the results can range from useless to deadly, since each animal metabolizes drugs differently.

Find out whether a horse metabolizes the drug or "nutrient" in the same way as the animal or person on which it was tested. Horses have a unique digestive system, monogastric (having one stomach, like humans) but also herbivorous (eating only plants, like a cow). A horse can manufacture many of the nutrients we humans need from our food because of his huge cecum. This fermentation vat is not quite as efficient as the cow's rumen, but it provides the horse with such nutrients as vitamins B_{12}, K, and C. The horse's unique digestive system has a profound effect on the way nutrients are processed in the body, and is one reason why we can't simply extrapolate dosages from other animals by weight alone.

What does all this mean in practical terms? Haven't people used certain products on their horses for years without ill effects and sometimes with wondrous results?

While many of the products do work, others act like a placebo for frustrated horse owners looking for a cure; still other horses would have recovered in the same way without the product's help. The safest route is to choose only products that have been tested on horses and whose makers have the data to back up their claims.

If you choose to use an untested product on your horse, here are some ways to stay on the safe side. First, use products that are time-tested; let other horse owners experiment on their horses first.

Second, request product literature and scientific studies from the manufacturer. Get your vet's help in evaluating a study you don't understand. Avoid products making outrageous claims or companies that refuse to send you information.

Third, be aware that any product sold as a feed supplement has not undergone drug testing. No matter what kind of testimonials or "research" the company quotes, true studies on the product's value have not been done. While some of these products are worthwhile, you must investigate further before you spend your money.

Finally, consult with your veterinarian to be sure that no negative side

Alternative
Medicine
and Therapy

effects have been reported for that product. Ask your veterinarian to find out the latest word on the effectiveness and safety of the product.

Every medication and nutrient is helpful when properly and knowledgeably used. We must balance our urge to find the miracle supplement with common sense. Don't believe outrageous claims, but ask questions and be ready to absorb new information with an open mind.

Alternative Therapy and Therapeutic Devices

"Physiotherapy" is the use of physical agents and methods to assist in rehabilitation or prevent injury. It includes the use of heat and cold, massage, hydrotherapy, and various medical devices, including electrotherapy, cold lasers, and ultrasound.

As a horse owner, you will be bombarded with advertisements for new therapeutic tools and equipment. The various devices can be quite expensive, and some are labeled For Veterinary Use Only, so you will probably rent one from your veterinarian if it is needed. Some are relatively harmless, others will help your horse, and a few could make your horse worse off than before. If you think that a machine is a safe alternative to drugs, recall that machines can also cause unseen harm.

Find out all that you can about a product before you spend your money, then use only what is appropriate for you and your horse. If a product seems too good to be true, it usually is. The safest approach is to have your veterinarian, trainer, and physical therapist or massage therapist work as a team with you to determine what is best for your horse.

Heat and Cold as Therapy

The simplest, cheapest, and often the finest forms of therapy are the use of heat and cold. While general guidelines are given here, ask your veterinarian's advice about your horse's specific injury.

Applying ice or running a cold hose over a sprain or strain is the best treatment for immediate relief. The drop in temperature reduces swelling and pain, and decreasing inflammation helps prevent worsening of the condition.

Cold therapy helps most during the first day or two after an injury, while the injury is still acute. Treat an old, chronic injury as acute if it flares up after exercise. Whether you use a cold wrap, a hose, or an ice boot, apply the cold treatment for about twenty minutes at a time, remove it for twenty to forty minutes, and reapply.

There are many different types of ice boots, whirlpool boots, gel packs, and the like that you can use. Make your own if you prefer (ice in a plastic bag), or experiment with commercial products to find one that is easy to use. Most refrigerant sprays and electric cooling devides do not provide adequate deep cooling.

After the second day, or when the inflammation is reduced, alternate applications of heat and cold to an injury. Heat will increase circulation and dilate blood vessels, while cold constricts the vessels and decreases swelling. Theoretically, the heat will stimulate blood flow and healing while the cold prevents excessive swelling afterward.

Chronic injuries are those lasting more than a week. Once an injury has become chronic, an increase in circulation through the use of heat may help healing.

There are several ways that you can apply heat. The simplest is through massage, which stimulates the circulation. Massage is ideal for soft tissue injuries, minor aches and pains. A good massage therapist might make the difference in winning or losing at top levels of competition.

You can apply a liniment or paint to the horse's legs for more heat. (See chapter 4.) Therapeutic ultrasound provides deeper heat. Heating pads, heat lamps, and diathermy (an electrical heat generator) all have the potential of dangerously overheating or burning the horse. Use these with extreme caution, and never leave the horse unattended.

Pin-firing is an older method of increasing the circulation. An electric iron makes small burns in a dot pattern over the leg. In theory, the procedure turns an old, chronic injury into a new, acute one that can go on to heal. In practice, the horse is put through a painful procedure that creates new scar tissue. The main benefit to the injury is that several months of rest are recommended after pin-firing. Try using the rest by itself instead.

Therapeutic Ultrasound

Ultrasound consists of high-frequency sound waves. Two types of ultrasound, diagnostic and therapeutic, are used in veterinary medicine. Diagnostic ultrasound creates a picture of internal organs. Your veterinarian might use it to visualize your mare's pregnancy or to check the condition of a bowed tendon.

Therapeutic ultrasound uses sound waves of a different intensity than does diagnostic ultrasound. These ultrasonic waves create heat when they pass through tissue. Ultrasound therapy, which is used to increase heat and circulation in chronic muscle and tendon injuries, creates heat deeper in the tissues than massage or liniments can.

Ultrasound therapy should not be used on infected tissues, and it must be used with care on bone because the vibrations created by sound waves will prevent a fracture from healing. Fresh (acute) injuries will also worsen if therapeutic ultrasound is applied.

Electrostimulation and
Electromagnetic Therapy

The concept of electrical or magnetic therapy is seductive. The machines look space-age and the theoretical results are astounding. Although most machines are sold with a For Veterinary Use Only label, they have found their way into many trainer's hands.

You'll need to do a bit of research before you can understand the complexities of electromagnetic therapy. (See appendix for references.) There are several machines with the terms *electro* or *magnetic* in their names, and they can be very different.

The uses and effects of electrical and magnetic devices depend on the wavelength and frequency of the energy emitted. Low-frequency devices include low-frequency magnetic field devices, transcutaneous electrical nerve stimulators (TENS), and muscle stimulators. Therapies using higher frequency include diathermy and cold lasers.

Veterinarians and doctors use low-frequency electromagnetic fields to help mend bone fractures. An electric current can be created using a magnetic wrap with a pulsed magnetic field or with electrodes placed on or implanted under the skin. These devices are also thought to help increase blood blow, provide heat, or relieve pain, but studies on those effects are scarce.

Manufacturers of a nonelectrical, nonpulsed magnetic pad claim that their devices increases blood flow without creating heat. Their studies are still pending.

The transcutaneous electrical nerve stimulator (TENS) is a device that applies an electrical current to electrodes on the skin to treat pain. Its well-proven effects are short-lived.

Muscle stimulators provide an electrical pulse to the muscle, causing it to contract involuntarily. These machines are used successfully in human medicine to condition muscles that have temporarily lost their nerve supply. They are said to help increase blood flow and maintain range of motion. After an injury, some muscles may not be used because of pain. Theoretically, a muscle stimulator keeps the muscle moving and prevents wasting due to disuse.

Most of the electrical devices are purported to relieve pain. In horses, this effect may not be desirable. Whatever the injury, it will worsen if the horse does not perceive pain and is allowed to exercise. However, some people feel that pain relief from using a device is preferable to pain relief from drugs. Be aware that some organizations ban the use of medical devices just as they ban certain drugs during competition.

It must be pointed out that side effects from using any of these machines are possible and as yet unknown. There has been very little work done with any of the electrical machines on horses. Moreover, few

Easy Health Care
For Your Horse

studies have been done on the health effects of machines on the people that are operating them. Research has been "pending" for years; ask manufacturers for results of their clinical studies.

If you choose to use one of these devices, be sure your horse's problem is accurately diagnosed and that you are using the right machine in the proper place. Be sure your veterinarian is familiar with the machine and with the general concepts of electrical therapy. Stop treatment if the problem worsens, does not resolve, or if your horse seems uncomfortable during treatment.

Laser Therapy

Lasers have gone from space-age theory to practical use. The LASER, an acronym for Light Amplification by Stimulated Emission of Radiation, is a device that produces electromagnetic radiation of particular wavelengths.

There are two basic types of lasers. Hot, high-power, or surgical lasers have a cutting or burning effect. The surgeon uses the laser to cut or remove tissues without touching them. The fine beam allows for extreme precision, even in small areas. The result is less tissue injury, less scarring, and more rapid healing than with traditional surgery.

Cold, soft, medical, or therapeutic lasers have a low-power beam that is used to treat muscle and bone injury or to stimulate acupuncture points. Two types of cold lasers are helium–neon and gallium arsenide (infrared). While they do not burn as the hot lasers do, therapeutic lasers can damage your eyes if you look into the beam.

Cold lasers are used to stimulate acupuncture points, to reduce pain, or to speed healing. Whether or not these effects occur is controversial. Far less research has been done with cold-laser therapy than with the surgical variety. Many of the studies that have been done are not considered valid by the medical and scientific community, so until more research is done, the use of therapeutic lasers must be considered experimental.

Acupuncture

Acupuncture is one of the world's oldest treatments. Few people doubt that acupuncture works. However, without consistent standards for evaluating and licensing acupuncturists, there is great potential for intentional and unintentional misuse of acupuncture. Beware of cure-all claims and proceed cautiously.

Acupuncture points can be stimulated with needles, a cold laser, electromagnetic stimulation, or hand pressure. No matter how it is performed, acupuncture should be done by a trained veterinary acupuncturist.

Acupuncture can be used to help reach a diagnosis or to relieve pain, but is not usually used to treat infections or cure diseases. As with all pain-relieving treatments, acupuncture should be used only after the cause of the pain has been found and treated. Pain relief alone should not be used as an indication of the horse's readiness to return to work. Most veterinary acupuncturists use acupuncture as one of many tools, integrating traditional medicine with acupuncture for the best results.

The American Veterinary Medical Association has recognized acupuncture as a valid procedure if it is performed by a person with advanced training. There is only one veterinary acupuncture organization, the International Veterinary Acupuncture Society (IVAS), which trains veterinarians in a course offered yearly in various parts of the country. The society can provide a list of veterinarians who have gone through this training. (See appendix.)

How to Investigate Something New

No matter how many treatments or new pieces of equipment we might mention, you'll continue to encounter new and different therapies and products. How can you determine whether they really work? How can you protect yourself from false claims, prevent further injury to your horse, yet still take advantage of new and better treatments?

First, recognize the difference between scientific studies and testimonials. Testimonials are quotes from "satisfied users" in which they claim wondrous results from using the product. Remember, any company can find someone to say what the company wants.

On the other hand, you'll find literature that bombards you with so much technical information that you're unable to ask the simplest question. Don't be impressed by big words or scientific baloney. Write to the company and ask it to explain precisely how, for example, its machine restores the ionic balance of the tissues, and ask for copies of the study showing how that makes your horse heal faster.

Stay away from a product or machine that seems to cure everything. If any product could truly do so, then your vet would be using it all the time and making a fortune. Look for products that list specific situations where they should or should not be used.

Ask your veterinarian about the product. If he or she is not familiar with it, ask for sources of further information. Look for information beyond that given to you by the company selling the product. Read everything you can find about any product or therapy.

Remember that hope will influence the outcome of your and other's use of a product. In human medical studies the placebo effect is quite strong; a pill with nothing in it cures a good percentage of patients.

When people tell you that a product worked well for their horses, get more information before you blindly use it on your own animal.

Finally, have your horse's problem thoroughly investigated and diagnosed by a veterinarian before any treatment is begun. Look for a veterinarian, trainer, and physical therapist or massage therapist who can work together for your horse's benefit. No problem can be accurately treated until it is identified, and no treatment works for every problem. If you choose an experimental therapy, be sure that you can afford it, that you're well aware of any known risks, and that you realize there may be unknown or unreported risks as well.

Today's accepted methods of treatment were among yesterday's experiments, but not all of those experiments resulted in useful treatments. If you keep an open mind and ask a lot of questions, you and your horse can make the most of new therapies and products.

Appendix

Sources of Further Information

Adams' Lameness in Horses, Fourth Edition
Ted S. Stashak, DVM, MS
Lea & Ferbiger, 1987
This is the classic text on equine lameness; it is written for veterinarians.

Beating Muscle Injuries for Horses
Jack Meagher, Sports Therapist
PO Box 713
667 Wethersfield Street
Rowley, MA 01969
A how-to book on massage therapy for horses that is written by a recognized expert in the field.

The Body Language of Horses
Tom Ainslie & Bonnie Ledbetter
William Morrow & Co., Inc., 1980

Explains why horses do what they do, and how you can use that knowledge to understand and solve behavior problems. Helps you learn to communicate with your horse.

Breaking Your Horse's Bad Habits
W. Dayton Sumner
A. S. Barnes and Co., Inc, 1976

Discusses common behavior problems, why they occur, and what to do about them.

Breeding Management & Foal Development
Equine Research, Inc., 1982
PO Box 9001
Tyler, Texas 75711

An excellent text that covers everything about breeding horses, from breeding farm design to mare and stallion management.

Clinical Electrotherapy
Roger M. Nelson & Dean P. Currier
Appleton & Lange, 1987

A technical book for those inclined to research the devices used in some types of physical therapy.

Drugs and the Performance Horse
Thomas Tobin
Charles C. Thomas Publisher, 1981
Springfield, IL

Discusses the actions, effects, and consequences of drug use in performance horses.

Equine Injury & Therapy
Mary Bromiley
Howell Book House, 1987

Written by a British equine physical therapist, this book discusses various injuries and types of physical therapy.

Equine Sports Therapy
Mimi Porter
Veterinary Data, 1990

Covers all aspects of equine physical therapy.

Feeding and Care of the Horse
Lon Lewis, DVM, PhD
Lea & Ferbiger, 1982

The classic nutrition text used by both veterinarians and horse owners.

Easy Health Care
For Your Horse

Grooming to Win
Susan E. Harris
Charles Scribner's Sons, 1977
Covers grooming for all types of competition.

Nutrient Requirements of Horses
National Research Council
National Academy Press
2101 Constitution Avenue NW
Washington, DC 20418
The ultimate reference to use when formulating a horse's ration. This booklet lists the nutrient content of most feeds and shows how to calculate what may be missing from the horse's diet.

Popular Nutritional Practices: Sense and Nonsense
Jack Z. Yetiv, MD, PhD
Dell Publishing, 1988
Although this book is written about human nutritional fads, it is just as applicable to the use of equine supplements. The reasons behind the use of various nutrients is clearly explained. This book is essential in helping you to understand the reality behind various products' claims.

Show Grooming: The Look of a Winner
Charlene Strickland
Breakthrough Publications
A how-to book for grooming your horse.

Tack Buyer's Guide
Charlene Strickland
Breakthrough Publications
This book thoroughly discusses and illustrates all types of tack.

Veterinary Pharmaceuticals and Biologicals
(Revised every other year)
Veterinary Medicine Publishing Co
9073 Lenexa Drive
Lenexa, Kansas 66215
A technical reference that lists all the medications approved for use in animals. Gives dosages, effects and side effects, indications and contraindications for various drugs, medications, dewormers, and vaccines.

Training and riding books are not listed because there are so many choices. Ask your trainer to recommend a book for your particular situation.

Associations

Contact these groups for further information. Ask about what they can offer in terms of publications, directories, and other assistance.

International Veterinary Acupuncture Society
Dr. Meredith Snader
2140 Conestoga Road
Chester Springs, PA 19425

This group instructs and certifies veterinary acupuncturists; they can give you a list of veterinarians who have gone through their course.

American Horse Shows Association, Inc.
220 East 42nd Street, Suite 409
New York, NY 10017-5806

The AHSA is the governing body for many competitive events. They publish the *American Horse Shows Association Directory*, a list of all committees, offices, and affiliated associations of the AHSA. They also publish a newsletter called *Horse Show*.

American Horse Shows Association
Drugs & Medications Control Program
3780 Ridge Mill Drive
Hilliard, OH 43026

Contact this office for information on drug testing and regulations.

American Horse Council
1700 K Street NW Suite 300
Washington, DC 20006

The AHC is a national trade association representing all horse-related interests. They publish the *Horse Industry Directory*, an essential reference that lists almost every horse group, association, publication, or resource that exists.

American Farrier's Association
4089 Iron Works Pike
Lexington, KY 40511

The AFA publishes the American Farrier's Journal; it also holds an annual convention and competition for farriers. This group tests and certifies farriers at various levels of expertise.

Equine Travelers of America, Inc.
PO Box NR-322
Arkansas City, KS 67005

Publishes the *Nationwide Overnight Stabling Directory*, a list of places you can stay overnight with your horse.

The United States Pony Clubs, Inc.
893 South Matlack Street #110
West Chester, PA 19382
A national group devoted to developing the riding skills of people under the age of eighteen. (Not limited to pony riders!)

Index

223

Index